Running Past Fifty

Running Past Fifty

Advice and Inspiration for Senior Runners

GAIL WAESCHE KISLEVITZ

FOREWORD BY AMBY BURFOOT

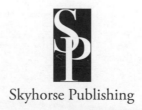

Skyhorse Publishing

Skyhorse Publishing books may be purchased in bulk at special discounts for sales promotion, corporate gifts, fund-raising, or educational purposes. Special editions can also be created to specifications. For details, contact the Special Sales Department, Skyhorse Publishing, 307 West 36th Street, 11th Floor, New York, NY 10018 or info@skyhorsepublishing.com.

Skyhorse® and Skyhorse Publishing® are registered trademarks of Skyhorse Publishing, Inc.®, a Delaware corporation.

Visit our website at www.skyhorsepublishing.com.

10 9 8 7 6 5 4 3

Library of Congress Cataloging-in-Publication Data is available on file.

Cover design by Tom Lau
Cover photo credit: iStockphoto

Print ISBN: 978-1-5107-3629-0
Ebook ISBN: 978-1-5107-3630-6

Printed in China

For Susan Sheets Brogan
Your smile, contagious laugh, and passion for life continue to
inspire me every day. You live on in all our hearts.

Contents

Foreword by Amby Burfoot   xi

Introduction   1

Profiles

Julio Aguirre   13

Amy Bahrt   19

Gordon Bakoulis   25

George Banker   31

Kathy Bergen   37

Witold Bialokur   45

Karen Bowler   51

Michael Brooks   59

Kevin Follett   67

Jeff Galloway   73

Julian Gordon   79

Harold Green   85

William Gross   91

Alisa Harvey   97

Sabra Harvey   105

Julia Hawkins   113

George Hirsch   121

Sid Howard 127

Robert Lida 133

Betty Lindberg 139

James Manno 145

Gerald Miller 151

Charles Milliman 157

Tom Perri 165

Kimi Puntillo 171

Bill Rodgers 175

Ed Rousseau 181

Alan Ruben 187

Drew Swiss 193

Kathrine Switzer 199

Kathryn Waldron 207

Ed Whitlock 213

Motivating Factors

Julia Chase 219

Brian Salzberg 225

Jonathan Mendes 229

James Austin 233

Jamie and Lynn Parks 239

Lessons Learned **243**

Advice from the Experts 253

Closing Remarks 263

Senior Events 267

Bibliography/Further Reading 269

Acknowledgments 271

Foreword

It's no coincidence that Gail Kislevitz and I recently found ourselves working on similar book projects at the same time—my *Run Forever: Your Complete Guide to Healthy Lifetime Running* and her *Running Past Fifty: Advice and Inspiration for Senior Runners*. In fact, it was almost inevitable.

We both began our running adventures in the 1970s, we've both reached retirement age, and neither of us has any intention of giving up the energy and vibrant good health that running has brought us for nearly fifty years. Writers research and write about the passions that permeate their lives, so we both turned naturally to the subject of lifetime running and runners.

And we're not alone. Around the globe, there are hundreds of thousands of other runners pushing back the boundaries of aging, fitness, running, and optimal health. I'm not sure there's much rhyme to us ancient marathoners, but we've got plenty of reason.

I often reflect on the differences between my father and me. He was a World War II vet whose happy-retirement dream included a summer evening, a beach, a sunset, a porch, a rocking chair, and a cold lemonade. He couldn't imagine more. He would be happy to just sit there and relax in the moment.

How am I different? In many ways, not so much. I'm also a fan of beaches, sunsets, porches, rocking chairs, and cold drinks, albeit ones that are stronger than lemonade. But here's the thing. I can't be content to just sit and rock. I also want to walk and run on the beach, and then plunge into the ocean. I want to move. I want to feel my arms, legs, and heart working in perfect synchrony. I want to get warm and sweaty, then cool and water-splashed. Because I know these simple pleasures will boost my evening enjoyment.

I know Gail and many others feel the same. We are the first generation in the history of Homo sapiens—literally the first ever; think about it—who want to stay fit and active all our lives. Why? Because we know how good it feels, and we don't ever want to relinquish that zest.

Once I was fast and loved being fast. Anyone who refuses to acknowledge the thrill of victory isn't being honest. Tell me I have a chance to win, and I will move mountains.

These days I no longer win. On a good day, I finish in the middle of the pack. On a bad day, I get lost in the rear. It doesn't matter. I don't run to collect medals and trophies. I run to enhance my life. And it works incredibly well.

At one point in my life, I sprinted the final blocks of the Boston Marathon as fast as I could, because one's Boston Marathon time was essentially the national pecking-order among US runners. Now I see Boston from an almost inside-out perspective, and find it incredibly refreshing and rewarding.

A block from the finish line, I slow to a walk. There's no need to hurry. I look skyward to give thanks and glance all around me to soak in the fantastic scene—sidewalk crowds screaming for every finisher, people leaning out of tall buildings to applaud, the gigantic Boston Marathon finish banner just ahead. Friends and family waiting to embrace me just past the finish line. I often tell fellow runners that "Every mile is a gift." This is never truer than at the end of the Boston Marathon. I want to fully appreciate every moment.

All the inspirational runners chronicled in this book have completely different stories and personalities, and yet we all share much. We also like to hang out together to talk about our training, our racing, our challenges, our sore muscles, and our future goals. Much is made in running circles of this "camaraderie." But what is it?

Most dictionaries define camaraderie as "mutual trust and friendship among people who spend a lot of time together." Sounds formal. It's not.

Runners frequently note that to be an elite athlete you must "choose your parents well." That's a reference to the substantial role that genetics play in elite performance. I believe, in addition, that we should "choose our friends well."

Once, health and fitness research mainly centered on the physiologic returns—better heart health, lower blood pressure, less diabetes, and the like. Now things are shifting. More and more, we are concerned with mental health, from depression to Alzheimer's. And guess what? Running is just as good at boosting emotional well-being as it is in promoting physical wellness. And emotional health is an absolutely central factor in the aging process. If you can stay mentally strong, you have a much better chance of staying physically strong.

Ultimately, that's why books like this one—and the runners you meet here—are so important. They will touch and positively influence every aspect of your life.

Gail and I often get together for one of our runs along the Eastern Connecticut shoreline. We'll scramble along some beaches, zigzag up a few hills, and seek out other low-density pathways. We have similar tastes in this regard. As we run, the conversation will flow easily. We'll discuss our training and race plans, of course. But we'll also check up on each other's kids, chat about enticing new travel adventures, discuss recent books and movies, and mull possible writing projects. The minutes and miles will fly past.

Before we know it, we will have covered six or eight or ten miles, followed by a brief frolic in Long Island Sound and a hearty bowl of oatmeal (with blueberries, walnuts, and maple syrup, of course). I can't imagine a more perfect morning.

We've done many a run like this. We have many more to come.

Amby Burfoot, *Runner's World* writer at large

Introduction

When you are a lifelong runner like I am, you can't imagine a day without running in it. The joys and benefits of a running life are something to be cherished and nurtured. When I first discovered running as a teenager in the sixties, it brought unbridled joy and an energy and empowerment I had never felt before. It became my best friend and stuck with me through thick and thin, boyfriend breakups, going off to college and being away from home for the first time, and helped me cope with grades and all-nighters. My running life continued to see me through marriage, graduate school, working, and giving birth to two kids.

Through the years, running has never let me down, never disappointed me, always lifted me up when I needed it. I never took it for granted and happily assumed we would grow old together. Well, now I have reached that age when my running life, although still joyous, also consists of avoiding injuries and trying not to relive or chase down personal bests from the past.

Denials about the aging process and the effects it has can sometimes trip us up as we age. We need new tools to help reset our running life and embrace the new goals that will help us to be the best we can be as we age.

The most important goal should be to run for life, to enjoy the running life for as long as we can. That's not meant to sound ominous, just realistic. Most of us beyond the age of fifty know that life is short and that we need to embrace every day. But it can be difficult to come to grips with the reality that age slows us down and makes us more prone to injuries. Little lessons become essentials, like the fact that recovery takes longer and becomes more important than when we were younger. Speed workouts need to be modified to emphasize quality over quantity.

And most of us are now assigned to the mid-pack in the starting-line corrals—an apt metaphor for where we are in our lifespan.

There is no shortcut through old age, but by running, we can turn back the clock, or at least slow its effect on the way we feel and look and stay healthy and fit. I'd like to feel that masters' runners are also changing the face of aging and what it means to be athletic at our age. We are not going quietly into old age. Don't even think about breaking out the rocking chair.

I started running when I was sixteen under cover of darkness, as girls were not encouraged to run. I loved the freedom it gave me, and I'll admit there was a little, "Don't tell me I can't do something" attitude. Now, more than fifty years later, running has enhanced my life and keeps me busy and fulfilled. As sixty-eight-year-old Sabra Harvey, a world-record-holding sprinter and grandmother, tells her kids, "Check with my race calendar before you ask me to babysit."

My new motto is, "Don't look back. Be happy with whatever tomorrow brings." My pursuit is to run endless miles and to enjoy running forever. I want to hear the slap of my shoes against the road, feel the breeze in my face, explore new roads, kick up some leaves, run through the first snowfall, and nod at the runners coming and going, knowing we share a secret. We understand that running isn't just a sport, a way to lose weight or to get some cardio in before going to the gym. It is our passion, our fervor, a force within us that in some cases keeps us alive. It flows through our veins like a life force.

The effects of running for me are so powerful that sometimes I can't explain it; I just feel it and know it and miss it when I am injured. As I age, I want my running to be my constant companion as it has been throughout my life. We will grow old together. And sometimes, on a perfect day when I go out for a run and nothing hurts and I feel the breeze at my back and the sun on my face and wear a mile-wide smile, I feel like that sixteen-year-old girl again out for her first run.

How I Became a Runner

Since most psychologists tell us we are defined by our past and our family upbringing, I'll share with you how I came to be a runner. I come from a family lineage steeped in the military. My grandfather served in World War I. My great-uncle, Admiral Russell Waesche, earned praise from President Truman for his stewardship during World War II. He was the first Coast Guard officer to achieve that rank. Ironically, one of the runners profiled in this book, James Manno, served under him during the war. When Pearl Harbor was attacked, my father was a senior at Dartmouth College and wanted to enlist in the Navy. The Dartmouth College president at that time, Ernest Hopkins, realized he would lose many of the college's young men to war, so he accelerated their curricula and shifted to a three-term, year-round schedule. Another runner profiled in this book, Jonathan Mendes, was in his class at Dartmouth. Dad graduated with his degree and entered the navy where he was assigned to the destroyer, the USS *Callaghan*.

While on a convoy in the Pacific, the USS *Callaghan* was attacked and sank with a loss of forty-seven crewmembers. She was the last Allied ship sunk by a kamikaze during the war. For twelve hours, my dad treaded water that was burning with oil residue and strafed by bullets. A strong swimmer, he gave his life preserver to another seaman who couldn't swim. I mention this because when I am dragging at mile 20 in a marathon, I think of him and what he went through during the war. After the war he returned home and married his Brooklyn sweetheart, Beatrice Maleady, and they started a family while he earned his law degree at Columbia.

I grew up in Oradell, New Jersey, one of four siblings: I have two older brothers and a younger sister. Growing up in the fifties, I was a tomboy, a term not used very much anymore. After school I quickly changed out of my Catholic school uniform and followed my two older brothers into the woods in our backyard to catch frogs and turtles. I tried to keep up with them as best I could. My little sister wasn't so lucky. Occasionally she was tied to a tree "to keep her safe." Our summers were spent in New London, Connecticut, on the shore of Long Island Sound, where we learned to swim, sail, and watch for shooting stars at night. It was idyllic. And such freedom. There was no schedule, programs to attend, or monitoring of clocks. And because it was a close-knit beach community where everyone watched out for one another, our parents didn't care where we were or what we were doing all day.

The sixties brought a change to our lives and a new emerging culture that would define not just us but our world. I switched from listening to Peter, Paul and Mary to the Beach Boys to Bob Dylan. Our generation was told to not trust anyone over thirty, and our music raged against age with lyrics such as, "What a drag it is getting old," sung by a twenty-four-year-old Mick Jagger. Or my favorite, "Will you still need me, will you still feed me when I'm sixty-four," sung by Paul McCartney when he was twenty-five. Or Simon and Garfunkel singing, "How terribly strange to be seventy."

School sports back then were mainly for boys. I watched my older brothers run cross country and track at River Dell High School and was envious. I watched them run through the woods in the fall, through snowstorms in winter and along the beach in the summer; they returned glistening with sweat, tired, but thrilled with themselves. I wanted that feeling. I wanted to push myself and test myself like they did. But there was no track or cross-country teams for girls. I could be a cheerleader or a flag twirler. I admit to trying out for both and being rejected. Recently, I pulled out my high school yearbook, graduating class of 1969. There under my picture in the graduation gown, long blond hair parted in the middle just like Joni Mitchell, were listed the following activities: Alternate Hawk (our school mascot; I never did get to wear the hawk outfit), Nurses Club (that had to be a typo), Pep Club, and Junior Prom Decorating Committee. No wonder my daughter thinks I was a nerd in school.

Not allowed to run on a team, I took matters into my own hands. On a summer night in 1967, I pulled on my Keds, took our golden retriever with me as a training partner, and went out for my first run. I didn't tell anyone. I ran around the block, probably less than half a mile, but it was enough to leave me tired and ecstatic. (To put things in perspective, it was the same year Kathrine Switzer was almost shoved off the course at the Boston Marathon by race director Jock Semple for the sole crime of being female.) I returned home transformed and in love with running. And that's how it all started. I never stopped, never looked back, never backed down.

I went to Boston College and lived in an apartment off Beacon Street, a few blocks from the Boston Marathon course. I walked to campus, a three-mile trek around the Chestnut Hill Reservoir. I could have watched Nina Kuscsik become the first female to officially win the Boston Marathon in 1972, but none of that was on my radar. I was just happy to get in a daily run around the reservoir or the Boston College track.

I continued running at graduate school at Michigan State University. I married my high-school sweetheart, and we lived in a tiny married-housing apartment off campus. The Michigan winters were brutal, but I used my running as a break from the long hours of study. Back in New

Jersey, I kept up my running and ran my first race, the New York Road Runners L'eggs Mini Marathon, in 1975.

I kept plodding along with my running through two pregnancies and working full-time. My husband and I would switch off who ran first when getting home from work or on Saturday mornings. It wasn't until the sudden death of my mother in 1987 that the thought of running a marathon crept into my head. She died too young, at sixty-seven. I was thirty-seven with two young kids who adored her. Everyone adored my mother. She was a bright light in my life and then the flame went out. My life came to a halt and I crawled into a deep hole to escape the pain of her loss. After two years of depression that resulted in anorexia, I knew I had to do something to shake the doom-and-gloom existence I was living. I turned to my running and decided to run a marathon. My family and friends thought the idea was ludicrous, even dangerous, but I knew better. I knew that running would save me. I knew that to run a marathon I would have to get healthy. I knew that I would have to train properly and think positively and fuel myself. On my long runs with my friend Ellen, I spoke about my mom in a manner that years of therapy never helped. I started to feel whole again.

When I ran that first marathon, I had a blast and knew I was going to make this a lifelong pursuit. Ellen and I talked and laughed for twenty miles. When the going got rough at mile 21, we stopped talking to save our energy and focus. That's when my mom appeared at my shoulder. I could feel her presence and hear her soothing voice as she guided me through those last few miles. So now, when I run a marathon, I dedicate those last few miles to my parents, who continue to guide me not only through marathons but through life.

"At Your Age . . ."

I'm beginning to hate those words. I recently went to a sports doctor for an injury. After he diagnosed me with a muscle tear, he gave me the rundown of just about everything in my body that is shrinking, thinning, shortening, turning gray, decomposing. He read me the riot act about eliminating speed workouts and not killing myself for a ribbon. "Just enjoy running," he went on. "Isn't that enough of a goal? At your age you should think about retiring from racing and marathons."

I mounted my protest. "You don't know anything about me or what I'm capable of," I said. "You're just looking at a number and making assumptions. What about the sixty-five-year-old women in my age division who are still running sub-seven-minute miles?" He looked at me as if he were about to address a petulant child. "Anyone running at that pace at that age is an outlier," he said.

I left the office in a state of ambivalence. On the one hand, he's right. I haven't run a seven-minute mile in years and know it is out of my reach. Bravo for the women out there, the Kathy Martins and other outliers who are doing it. On the other hand, why shouldn't I keep trying and training to be the best I can be? Push myself to the point of depletion but not injury? Know that I gave it my all, whatever pace that may be? I can live with that. But I won't go back to that doctor again.

Who We Are

The 2017 US Census Bureau data shows seniors increasing faster than younger populations. According to the 2017 data, the nation's median age rose from 35.3 years on April 1, 2000, to 37.9 years on July 1, 2016. The baby-boom generation is largely responsible for this trend. And many of them are runners.

In the year 2000, people over sixty-five represented 12.4 percent of the population—a number expected to grow to 19 percent of the population by 2030. This rapid growth is due to the aging of the baby-boom generation.

People sixty-five years or older numbered 46.2 million in 2014 (the latest year for which data is available), and many of them are runners. Some of us picked up the sport during the first running boom in the seventies, inspired by Frank Shorter's gold-medal marathon performance at the 1972 Munich Olympics. Others came to the sport late in life, like 102-year-old Ida Keeling of New York, who became the first woman in history to complete a 100-meter race at the age of one hundred, in April of 2016. Her time was 1:17.33, and she later improved her 100-meter world record for one-hundred-year-old women to 59.80 seconds. Keeling started running at age sixty-seven and isn't slowing down.

According to the 2017 Running USA annual report on race statistics, masters' age groups at races reflect this population trend. The TCS New York City Marathon, the world's largest marathon with more than 50,000 finishers, is a prime example: the report found that 49 percent of the finishers were masters (forty years old and above), up from 48 percent in 2014. At the 2018 Brooklyn Half-Marathon, the largest half-marathon in the United States, 44 percent of the runners were masters. Another trend at marathons is that the top fifty finishers in the sixty-and-up age divisions are significantly faster than those in the past. And in a statistic that many never saw coming, 59 percent of race entrants are female.

Thank Goodness for Age-Division Classifications

With the help of Ken Stone, I tracked down a brief history of how we came to be masters runners. Ken is a wealth of knowledge and is eager to share it and spread the word. He keeps a blog, masterstrack.blog, which is a cornucopia of facts and statistics about masters track and field. He also helped write the book *Masters Track and Field: A History* by Leonard Olson (2010). As documented in the book, David Pain, a runner and lawyer in La Jolla, California, and Augie Escamilla, a member of the San Diego Track Team, along with Les Land, director of the San Diego Invitational track and field meet, held a meeting in early 1966 to discuss a mile event for men over forty. Pain proposed calling it "the Masters Mile." On June 11, 1966, fourteen entrants, men aged forty to sixty, ran the outdoor mile. The winner was forty-four-year-old Jim Gorrell, who ran a 4:47. The event became so popular, masters' mile events began popping up all over the country. Pain credits the San Diego Track Club as being crucial to the evolution of masters' athletics.

The first US National Masters Track and Field championships took place in July of 1968. Masters athletes from across the country attended, including Jim Hartshorne, forty-four, a professor at Cornell, who won the mile in 4:50 and was instrumental in bringing masters miles in open meets to upstate New York. In his introductory remarks before the event, Pain stated: "Senior runners are beginning to prove that a mature individual can be in superb physical condition . . . Champion athletes of past years may once again appear and compete. Younger men will be encouraged to continue in competition beyond the age at which athletes customarily compete."

As I scrolled down the list of winners from that first national track and field meet in 1968, one name jumped out at me: John A. Kelly, age sixty, came in third at the marathon event in 3:04. The winner was Richard Packard, forty, who won in 2:48. Another Boston Marathon familiar name, John Lafferty, fifty at the time of the national track and field meet, who ran the Boston Marathon five times between 1949 and 1953, placing second in 1951, ran the three-mile and six-mile event and won both. I asked Stone why the marathon was part of a track and field event. His response was that the marathon event boosted attendance. The marathon has since been dropped from USATF Masters Track and Field meets.

Women were not part of the masters' movement at first. Three decades after that first Masters Mile in 1968, Pain apologizes: "I am mortified that we did such a sexist thing," he says. "It's just an example of the conditions that prevailed." Subsequent events included women.

Why start at age forty? Pain was forty-four at the time he conceived of the masters category and picked forty as a starting point. Women could enter the masters' category at thirty-five, because Pain thought that wives and girlfriends were generally five years younger than their male counterparts. A subsequent ruling had both male and female masters' track and field categories start at age thirty-five. Olson's book is filled with anecdotal tidbits that runners will find both humorous and interesting.

Moving along to the masters' category in road racing, the timing was ripe for RRCA to start forming masters' age categories. And to be honest, back in the early 1960s, there were more track and field events than road races. Gary Corbitt, son of legendary ultrarunner Ted Corbitt, has his father's journals and history books. Ted was president of RRCA in 1960, and Gary has a cadre of logs and journals and issues of *Footnotes,* the RRCA publication.

Gary sent me some RRCA archives. At the eighth annual meeting of the RRCA, in April of 1965, one of the items of business was to create a masters and sub-masters program for age categories thirty-five to thirty-nine, forty to forty-four, forty-five to forty-nine, and sixty and over. Sara Mae Berman, who unofficially ran the 1970 Boston Marathon in 3:05, drew up plans for a women's RRCA auxiliary. Women's and men's masters' races appeared in Baltimore in late 1964.

It would take two more years for the RRCA to hold their first masters' event, a National Cross Country Championship for men over forty, held at Catonsville, Maryland, in October of 1967. Jim Hartshorne once again proved his mettle by winning the event. A second RRCA Cross Country Championship for men over forty was held at Catonsville on October 6, 1968, with divisions for forty to forty-nine, fifty to fifty-nine, sixty to sixty-nine, and seventy-plus.

I asked Ken Stone what the appeal was for masters track and field. "The camaraderie and the social aspect is the main attraction," he said. "It's the chance to act crazy as kids or competitive as the young guns.

We've earned the right to do whatever we want." Competition plays an important part as well. When he attends senior meets, Stone says he can see it in the eyes of the ninety-year-old sprinters who are going head-to-head and giving it their all. "They are hammering to the finish," he adds. "When they compete, it's no-holds-barred, but once they finish, they're embracing one another and sharing laughs." The growth in masters' meets like the Huntsman Games, the National Senior Games, and the World Games supports Stone's theory that masters' track and field athletes are looking for events for competition and the social aspect of getting away for a few days. Reunions are held; friendships are forged. Expectations and behavior that can be intimidating at open events are cast aside, and the vintage skimpy track shorts and singlets come out. Hobbling around afterward with bags of ice taped to knees and ankles, anywhere it hurts, is the norm. The conversations trend around medical issues, who lost a spouse (or has a new one), who has a new injury or a new hip. Spouses and doctors fall into the same category: either they are in agreement about competing and enjoying the process, or they are left out.

The Beat Generation novelist Jack Kerouac sums up the adventurous spirit of masters athletes when he wrote in *On the Road*: "Nothing behind me, everything ahead of me."

Age-Graded Scoring

Another milestone in masters running is age-graded scoring. I love this as much as I love age divisions. Age-graded scoring, a handicap based on age, allows all individuals within a race to be scored against one another. That is done by first comparing the individual's finish time at that particular race distance to an "ideal" or best time achievable for that individual's age and gender. Age-graded scoring utilizes statistical tables to compare the performances of athletes at different distances, in different events, and against athletes of either gender and of any age.

Developed in 1989 by WAVA, World Association of Veteran Athletes (now WMA, World Masters Athletes), age-grading is best explained with an example given on the website runraceresults.com: Let's say a fifty-five-year-old male runs a marathon in 3:00:27. He would receive an age-graded score of 80.21 percent. That's because, according to the age-graded scoring tables, the "ideal" finish time for a fifty-five-year-old male is 2:24:22, and that's about 20 percent faster (about thirty-six minutes) than our fifty-five-year old ran. No matter how old you get, your age-graded score or "performance percentage" will be judged against the standard for your current age within your gender. WAVA developed the following broad "achievement levels" for use with age-graded scoring. A score within each range indicates the level of performance achieved by an athlete.

100 percent = approximate world-record level
90 to 99 percent = world class
80 to 89 percent = national class
70 to 79 percent = regional class
60 to 69 percent = local class

What Really Happens to Us as We Age

I look in the mirror and feel pretty good. I'm holding up well, I say to myself. There are signs of aging I can't ignore such as the gray hairs (which are meticulously covered by my hair colorist) and that awful dry skin from loss of collagen, gravity, and too many summers baking on the beach in the hot sun. It makes me cringe to think what I did to my skin back then. I can't reverse any of that, but I now wear sunscreen every day and a hat. I try not to run between 10:00 a.m. and 2:00 p.m. in the summer, when the sun is at its hottest. Along with the physical breaking down of our body parts, the one aspect of aging that is actually a good thing is that we know our days are numbered. We can clearly see the downhill. I say that's a good thing because it makes us realize we must not waste a precious day. In John Leland's book, *Happiness Is a Choice You Make* (2018), he interviews people eighty-five and above on what makes them happy in life. A metro reporter for the *New York Times,* Leland found that those he interviewed don't worry about common distractions that may bother younger people because at a certain age those issues just aren't that important. It's a good lesson for anyone but especially for aging runners who don't want to give up their PRs or are afraid they might look foolish in skimpy shorts and singlets. No one cares! Get over yourself. Look foolish; act foolish. Focus your energies on what makes you happy.

Bone Health: Bone Mass/Density

Bone mass, the product of bone volume and bone density, peaks at about age thirty. At menopause, women experience a rapid increase in bone loss for as long as ten years before it normalizes. Clinicians used to be taught in medical school that bone density is the gauge for assessing bone strength. In recent years, the idea of bone strength has moved beyond density alone. Bone density can be misleading, as even a good density report does not necessarily mean that fractures are unlikely. In fact, bones can be dense yet brittle. I was diagnosed with osteopenia at my most recent bone-density test. I thought female runners were protected from osteoporosis, but I was wrong. So now I take really big calcium pills and worry about getting a stress fracture.

Bone strength or bone quality is what makes a bone resistant to fractures. Most runners know that running builds strong bone health. Wolff's law (developed by the German anatomist and surgeon Julius Wolff in the nineteenth century) states, "Bone in a healthy person or animal will adapt to the loads under which it is placed. In healthy people, bones respond to stress by reforming to better handle that stress." For runners, that means the weight-bearing bones of the legs, pelvis, and spine tend to be stronger than the same bones in inactive people.

Muscle Mass

Muscle strength tends to peak in our late twenties and starts to decline in our late thirties. The loss of muscle mass happens at the rate of about 10 percent per decade while muscle strength, the ability to generate force, declines even more dramatically.

What can we do about this? According to Dr. Wendy Kohrt, a professor in the Division of Geriatrics at the University of Denver, the good news is that in general, older people's bone density, aerobic capacity, muscle strength, and cardiovascular fitness can adapt to exercise with the same relative improvements as healthy young adults do. Of course, we cannot stop the aging process. Bone loss cannot be prevented, but being physically active may slow age-related bone loss. Dr. Kohrt established the IMAGE research group—Investigations in Metabolism, Aging, Gender, and Exercise—at the University to continue research in this area. She firmly believes that staying active is the best way to attack aging. "Being active gives you more reserve—in essence, it buys you time," says Kohrt.

Reset the Goals

To avoid a dreaded PW (personal worst), we have to reset our goals. Maybe now is the time to compete against that toughest competitor: yourself. If you give it everything you've got and leave nothing on the course except some spit, sweat, and tenacity, you have achieved your goal. If world-class runner Kathy Martin can do that, the rest of us should be able to do the same. At sixty-eight, Martin has set numerous world and American records, but she finds the training getting tougher, and it's harder to maintain her rankings. "Records are meant to be broken, so I enjoy them while I have them and move on," she says. "I just switch my thought process and start every day realizing how blessed I am."

If you already run just for the pleasure of getting in a daily work-out, you may be ahead of the game. Regardless of the pursuit—a medal, or a time out from the day's stresses—running is a gift that needs to be nurtured, respected, and loved. Treat it well and you will enjoy running many, many miles throughout a long life.

Julio Aguirre

DOB: June 16, 1946

Residence: Perth Amboy, New Jersey

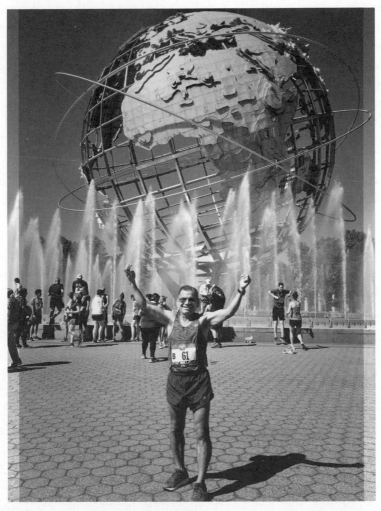

Julio Aguirre

Everyone Loves Julio.

When Julio Aguirre shows up for our interview, he is dressed in a dark blue suit and tie, looking dapper with a mischievous glint in his eye, as if he was about to share a secret. He is beyond charming. I knew this interview would be different from others and that I was in for a treat.

When I called him, he said he would prefer to meet in person as his English is not so good and he liked meeting people. I was familiar with his extraordinary running career, as he has won his age division thirteen times at the prestigious New York Road Runners (NYRR) Club Night that honors its top runners by age group. Although I knew of him and how the crowds cheer loudly for him at every race, I didn't know his story until we sat down together. I now have the utmost respect for Aguirre not only as a very accomplished runner, whose achievements include completing sixty-five marathons, but also as a humble person who has faced extreme challenges in his life and is on top of the world at age seventy-two.

Julio Aguirre was born in Ecuador in 1946, one of six kids. His father died when he was very young and the family lived in poverty. "I was a street kid," he explains. "I sold anything I could find on the street to make money for food." Although poor, his mother insisted that he go to school. She hoped that an education would be his ticket out of poverty, and her hunch was right. Aguirre found that he was smart enough to get good grades and be the top student in his class. That drive to excel, to be the best, would serve him later in life.

He became a high-school math teacher. But in a plot right out of a romance novel, he fell in love with one of his students; she was seventeen, he was twenty-five. He quit his job so they could continue their relationship. After she graduated, she moved to the United States, promising to return for him. She didn't return, but she sent him $800 to join her in New York. Excited to be reunited, he plotted his entry to the United States: he would first fly to Mexico City and then make his way to the US border in California. This was in 1977, and Aguirre had no papers or passport, so he would have to cross the border illegally. As he went through customs in Mexico City, nervous and excited, he revealed to the agent that he was carrying $800 in cash. What happened next is right out of the plot of a thriller: as he was en route in a cab to the bus depot where he'd get a bus to the border, two cars slammed into his cab and masked gunmen jumped out and demanded his money. Stunned and scared, Aguirre handed over the money and was left at the side of the road. Witnesses to the scene helped him out and gave him enough money to get to the border crossing.

As Aguirre tells the story, I'm on the edge of my seat. I can't imagine that this well-dressed man, beloved by all runners in the New York area, and a legend in his country, had such a gripping past.

It took him two weeks to cross the border with a "coyote," always on alert for border guards. With little food or water, he lost seventeen pounds during the journey. When he finally made it to Tijuana, the coyote put him in the trunk of a car for the six-hour ride to Los Angeles. His girlfriend wired more money for a train ticket from Los Angeles to New York City, a four-day journey, and all he could afford to eat was bananas. But it was all worth it when his love met him at Penn Station in Manhattan. Two weeks later they were married. Three months later he received his green card.

He was happily in love but didn't speak a word of English and had to take menial jobs. Over time, he became depressed and lonely, missing his family back in Ecuador. "I came from a professional background in my country, and here I was sweeping floors and pushing carts around," he says. After thirteen years, living in a basement apartment in Queens, desperately trying to support three kids, he found his life slipping into a dark hole and he felt there was no escape. He started drinking and smoking and his days got darker. His marriage crumbled and after thirteen years, his wife took the kids back to Ecuador.

"I didn't know who I was any longer," Aguirre says. "I was so miserable I just wanted to die." He started drinking with his friends every weekend. One day he and his friends went into Central Park to drink and after a night of it, he passed out. "I woke up and saw all these people running," he exclaims. Apparently, he woke up to see a NYRR race going past him in Central Park. It brought back memories of the time he won a 5K in high school. Aguirre is not a religious man, but that morning, seeing that race was an epiphany. "I felt something stir inside, and I wanted to run," he recalls.

The next day he started jogging in Flushing Meadow Park. Because of his drinking and smoking he didn't get far at first, but he kept at it every day, going a little farther with each jog. And little by little he gave up smoking and drinking. One year later, in 1992, at age forty-five, he entered a 5K and ran 22:13, a 7:10-per-mile pace, and placed thirteenth in his age division. He was euphoric. "I knew I had a lot of work to do to get to first place for my age, and I was up for it," he says. Three weeks later he ran a 10K at a 6:56 pace. He trained on his own, and with steely determination he moved up in the ranks until he was winning his age group. He ran nineteen races that first year. Three years after his first 5K, he was a nominee for Runner of the Year in his age division. He didn't win that year, but he could taste it. He knew he needed a team and a coach to improve his times and joined the West Side Runners. His running, and his life, started to blossom.

In 1994, healthy, athletic, and now working as a janitor, he went back to Ecuador to visit his family. He made amends with his former wife and his kids, spent time with his own family, and he met a new woman and fell in love. This time it was he who went back to America and she stayed behind. Two years later she appeared at his front door, and they got married. She encouraged him to go to Queens College and take English classes, to apply for citizenship, and to get a driver's license and a car so he could travel to his races. She stood at finish lines cheering for him. "I felt blessed, I was so happy," Aguirre says with a smile. And slowly he became a New York running legend.

Now everyone knows Julio. Whether it's his charm, his smile, his outgoing demeanor, or all of them combined, he became an icon at the races. That probably had something to do with the fact that he always wears a singlet and shorts, even in sub-zero weather. "It makes me run faster," he says with a grin.

Ten years ago, while winning yet another NYRR Runner of the Year award, Aguirre was approached by Gary Muhrcke, winner of the first New York City Marathon in 1970. Muhrcke, the founder and owner of the Super Runners Shop chain of running stores, heard his life story and, moved by his grit, offered him a job selling running shoes. Aguirre put the same determination and dedication into his job that he does with everything in his life, and soon he was the number-one salesperson.

Don't be lulled into thinking that Aguirre's charming persona carries over to the starting line. He is fiercely competitive. "When I don't win, I can't sleep," he admits. "When I get beaten, I work harder and that person never beats me again." His grueling training schedule leaves him injured at times. When he trained for the Staten Island Half at age fifty-three, the week leading up the race looked like this:

Monday: 10 miles in 1:04
Tuesday: 10 miles in 1:03
Wednesday: 10 miles in 1:02
Thursday: 10 miles in 1:01
Friday and Saturday: rest
Sunday: half marathon in a PR of 1:19:43

"Sometimes I kill myself in my workouts, but I have to," says Aguirre. "If I'm not working my hardest, someone will beat me."

In 2002, while "killing himself" doing 400-meter intervals, Aguirre nearly did kill himself. After the workout, he felt overly tired and had trouble walking home. When he got there, he collapsed in the hallway. His wife rushed him to the hospital, where he was diagnosed with a heart attack. Clots in his leg had traveled into his heart, and he was fitted with a stent. He spent fifteen days in the hospital, and the doctors advised him to give up running. He didn't. A week after he'd recovered enough to go home, he snuck out and jogged around the block. He kept this up, and a few months later, he won his age group at a half marathon. "I told a little white lie to my wife," he says with a smile. "I told her I was going to watch the race, not run it. I'm not going to sit back and watch my life go by, clots or no clots."

I don't think his wife was fooled.

The clots in his leg continue to plague him. His doctor says he is taking a risk every time he races. His wife worries about him and tells him he doesn't need any more medals to prove himself. In 2013, the problem reared its nasty head again. His body swelled and his running suffered. He took two years off to get them under control. "I hated those two years," Aguirre says emphatically. "I did a few test runs at a twelve-minute pace and wondered whether I'd ever make a comeback." He did. In 2018, he was once again named Runner of the Year in his age division at NYRR's Club Night. He has sworn off doctors. At this writing, he is keeping up a consistent 7:07 pace in races.

How does he do it? Aguirre is the first to say he doesn't do anything special. He has no special diet, he doesn't stretch, and he barely drinks water. (In his first twenty-four marathons, he didn't drink anything.) Why does he do it? "Running saved my life," he explains. "If I hadn't seen that race in Central Park that morning almost thirty years ago, God knows where I would have ended up. Probably dead." He admits to being a running addict. "I can't sleep if I haven't run. If there ever comes a time when I can't run, I would rather die."

Aguirre eats, sleeps, and lives for running. He can click off his race times and stats like reciting the alphabet. Now that he is getting older, he has to reset his goals and no longer looks for a personal best. "I just try to better my time from the previous year," he says. "That keeps me challenged."

Everyone knows Julio. He reminds me of the cult joke about a guy named Benny who knows everyone. One day a friend bets him $1,000 that he doesn't know the pope. So they go to the Vatican. Next thing you know, Benny's standing with the pope on the balcony overlooking Vatican Square, and his friend is shocked. But in a double shock, he hears a guy in the crowd say, "Who's the guy standing next to Benny?"

As if he is reading my mind about that joke, Aguirre tells me about a recent race expo where he stood in line to get an autograph from Bill Rodgers, one of his heroes whom he had never met. With just a few people remaining in front of him, a security guard comes over and tells him that the time is up and he has to leave, that Bill isn't giving any more autographs. Aguirre is disappointed but always the gentleman, he starts to leave. At that point, Bill looks up and sees him and says to the guard, "Oh, that's Julio. He can stay."

Aguirre knows he is lucky to be running at this level in his seventies. "I do feel I am beginning to take my age into account and try not to run over my ability," he says. "But I do want to win. My running life is the only life I know."

That's not quite true. Aguirre has another side to him. He has read all the classics and writes and recites poetry. He is very proud of his kids. One daughter has her PhD in English; the other is a teacher. His son works in real estate. His eleven-year-old grandson is already winning races and his four-year-old granddaughter isn't far behind. When he speaks about his kids, he tears up. In 2014, he was awarded the Ecuador Medal of Honor for International Sports Activity, presented by the country's president. When he tells me all this, it isn't boasting or bragging. It's from the heart and I can see the pride in his eyes.

Throughout our interview he hadn't stopped talking. He's like an excited kid who wants to tell you all about his amazing day and make you a part of it. But when I ask him to sum up his life, he pauses, leans back, and takes a minute before answering. "I'm not a religious man but I do believe in fate. There's a reason running came into my life and I need to honor that."

Aguirre is not a role model for aging runners. He takes risks that could derail his running or worse, be life-threatening. He needs to win. When asked if he could get to a point where he enjoys running for just the pleasure of an easy outing, he replies: "The thought of running for pleasure is yet to cross my mind. At this point in my life, the main objective is not to win, but to always win. My winning spirit is the main factor of my motivation."

Amy Bahrt

DOB: March 31, 1951

Residence: Manhattan, New York

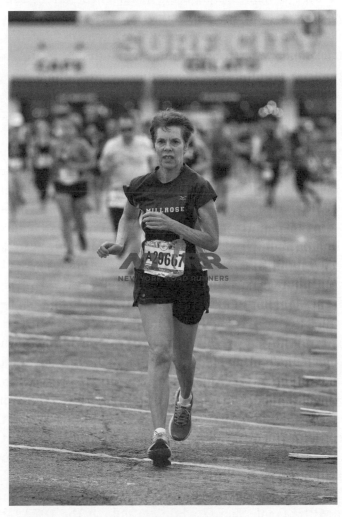

Amy Bahrt

"Running is Part of my DNA."

Amy Bahrt is realistic about how aging has affected her more than fifty years of running. She's not as fast as she was but can still place in her age division. She thinks of herself as an athlete but not a great one. What she has is the desire and passion for pursuing a sport that was once restricted for women but was there for the taking for the ones who had guts and determination. She describes herself as an everywoman, someone that any Average Jane can relate to. Her teammates at Millrose can attest to that but also to the fact that Bahrt's self-effacing manner belies a tough competitor.

Amy Bahrt grew up in River Edge, New Jersey, a town seven miles from the George Washington Bridge and access to New York City. In grammar school, she loved running the dash and beating the boys. Although she showed talent, in the 1960s girls were not allowed to compete on track or cross-country teams. So she took running into her own hands and ran around football fields, neighborhood streets, anywhere she could. "People stared but so what?" says Bahrt.

I went to high school with Bahrt at River Dell Regional High School in River Edge, New Jersey. She was one of the cool kids. Her parents were both artists, and her dad had a studio in Manhattan. For her sixteenth birthday, while other girls were having tea parties, Bahrt's dad took a group of kids into Manhattan for a sleepover in his photography studio. She and I were casual friends, but I wish we knew each other better because years later we discovered that back in high school we were both secretly running on the same back streets.

What drew Bahrt to running was the solitude. "I loved watching the guys run cross country, so I just did what they did, but undercover," says Bahrt. In college, at the Rhode Island School of Design, she ran up and down the hills of Providence and around the Brown soccer field. Her roommate had an old pair of Nike trainers that were worn out and gave them to her. As she recalls, "They were paper-thin, like running in flip-flops, but they were my first pair of running shoes!"

After graduating from college she moved to New York City and pursued her running. She became a regular on the path around the Jacqueline Kennedy Onassis Reservoir in Central Park. She joined Bob Glover's running class to learn proper form and training techniques. "I was inspired by Frank Shorter who won gold at the 1972 Olympics," states Bahrt. She also joined New York Road Runners. Back then, there were more males than females on the running scene and add to that the fact that she was a die-hard Rangers' fan, Bahrt became one of the boys.

Running became her focus. She joined a running club, and determined to learn the history of her newfound sport, she devoured everything she could about running. She went to see *Marathon Man,* thinking it was a movie about running. "That was a huge mistake. I couldn't go to the dentist for years after seeing that movie," she laughs. She started to notice changes in herself. She lost weight, became an extrovert. She found a whole new life, a cross-section of interesting, outgoing friends, a bit eccentric and crazy, but in a good way. A friend took her to a Millrose Game at Madison Square Garden where she was fascinated by the racing and competition. She met Fred Lebow, Kurt Steiner, Joe Kleinerman, Allan Steinfeld, and Ted Corbitt, all founders of NYRR. She was also inspired by the female pioneers of running such as Joan Benoit, Mary Decker Slaney, Nina Kuscsik, Kathrine Switzer, Grete Waitz, and Gillian Horovitz. "These ladies were so tough, yet gracious and fearless," adds Bahrt.

"I wanted to take my running to the next level and started training seriously," she adds. Her first race was the Perrier 10K in March of 1982. Her second race was the now iconic all women's L'eggs Mini 10K. She took a friend new to running to the event and she insisted they eat a huge breakfast to fuel up for the race. "I remember eating stacks of pancakes, eggs and bacon, even dessert," recalls Bahrt. "Of course I felt like vomiting all through the race. What did I know?"

She started volunteering at races, becoming part of the still-blossoming running scene in New York City. Her first marathon was the 1985 New York City Marathon, and she was one of just a few women. Statistics for that year show 13,270 men and just 2,467 females. Her parents came in from New Jersey to watch the race. "I didn't know anything about running a marathon. I ran next to a woman who wore a leopard-print bikini. My dad was gushing over the bikini gal but had no recollection of me!"

Now totally hooked on running and racing, she went to running camp in the summers and joined the Millrose Running Club. She started placing well in her age division and became noted among the serious runners in New York. But running in the 80s was still a male-dominant field. Bahrt recalls going to a race in Westchester and being harassed by a group of male runners challenging her right to be there. Later on, they became friends and the men changed their behavior toward Bahrt recognizing a kindred spirit.

During her forties and fifties, Bahrt ran with a passion she never knew possible. In her forties, she maintained an average 7:15-per-mile pace for races of under 15K. In her fifties, that slowed to 8:30 per mile, which she chalks up to menopause. But she still ran two or three marathons a year. Boston and New York were her favorite marathons. An old-school runner, she never got into the habit of stretching but she didn't suffer injuries.

All that changed in her sixties. Bahrt became chronically injured. When she finishing the 2014 Boston Marathon, she felt a pain in her knee but chalked it up to having just run 26.2 miles. By the time she got back to New York, she couldn't bend her knee. She went to an orthopedic doctor—a non-runner—who diagnosed her with acute osteoarthritis of the knee and told her she would never run again. Her first reaction after hearing the outcome was, "I'm going to either kill myself or him."

The doctor frustrated her in many ways, not just the diagnosis and dire warning of never running again. "I felt he looked at my age (sixty-three) and the fact that I was female and discounted me," she says. "He was not sympathetic to me as a runner or that it was a vital part of my life. He basically had no clue as to how important running was to me." A few weeks later she went to a recommended sports orthopedic who came up with the same diagnosis but suggested that she start physical therapy to see if it would help. A path to recovery had opened up.

A few months into her therapy she underwent SYNVISC knee shots, an injection that supplements the fluid in the knee to help lubricate and cushion the joint. She received one shot a week for three weeks, but the relief never came. Ultimately, she had to quit running for almost three years and spent time and money looking for the right treatment. "It was like a death for me," explains Bahrt. "All the things I had in common with my friends and peers were put on hold. I wasn't a part of the running scene anymore. Sure, I could have volunteered and cheered for my friends but that would only make me feel worse. It was a self-imposed prison sentence." During the three years of various treatments, she had a few good comebacks but always relapsed. It was a constant one-step forward, two-steps back cycle. Whenever she stopped the latest form of therapy, the knee pain returned.

Although she wasn't competing any longer, she still checked out the race results. She knew her times were no longer at the top of the heap. "I had to accept the fact that I probably wasn't ever going to get back to that level," she says. "We can't be fast and win forever. I had great years of racing and I'm not going to start making excuses for slower times."

In 2017, she tried another form of shots, Orthovisc, one shot a week for four weeks, and this time supplemented the shots with cross-training to build up the supporting muscles around the knee. She started with deep-water running, which she is a huge fan of and does it three times a week. She added Pilates and other kinds of strength training to her regime. "Physical therapy is a full-time job," she laments. "Between my full-time job and the therapy, I had no time left in the week." But this time the shots worked and her knee pain subsided.

During the years when she couldn't run she noticed small changes in her body. "I gained weight, my muscles atrophied, and I was sad all the time," she says. "People talk about muscle memory but I have to tell you, my muscles didn't remember a thing when I started running again. It was like being a baby and learning to walk."

By February of 2017, her new recovery treatment of the shots plus strength training was working and she saw results. She made a pact with herself to run the 2017 Philadelphia Marathon. She kept it a secret, not telling even her closest friends. "It was important to me to run another marathon to prove that I was back on track," she explains. "If I have to crawl, I'll finish this marathon." She cut back on her usual marathon training miles, logging 30 a week, (down from 55) and ran every other day. She took more time to warm up and cool down. She signed up for the Brooklyn Half Marathon in May of 2017 as a test of her endurance but didn't tell a soul, not even her teammates. She started at the back of the corrals, not wanting to see anyone or draw attention to the fact that she was there. She ran a steady pace, just happy to be logging the miles without pain and placed third in her age division. In her self-effacing manner, she says of the race: "I finished with the fanny pack and selfie-stick crowd but had a blast. Seems that everyone in my age division is also succumbing to injuries and age." Running the half-marathon gave her confidence about completing the marathon.

In November of 2017, she ran the Philadelphia Marathon. I emailed her before she left and she was nervous. On race day, the winds were howling, with gusts of 45 mph. A runners' advisory went out. Bahrt remained steadfast even as trees fell in front of her. Here is how she described her comeback marathon: "There were buckets of rain before the start and a gale headwind from mile seven on. I felt like I was strapped on to a rocket ship, or a leaf blower. It wasn't pretty and at times it was ridiculous. I saw two trees go down—one split before my eyes. No clocks, no valid mile markers—and I did not see a time at the finish."

But she ran steady and hard and finished in 4:30, placing first in her age group and qualifying for Boston 2019. Bahrt is back.

Despite her well-run race, she says her new goal is to run for life instead of running for competition. "I would do anything in the world to keep running forever," she says. "Running is a part of my life. Whether I am racing, doing a casual run with a friend or on the injured list, I define myself as a runner. It is who I am in my heart and soul."

It took a lot of hard work and pushing herself for Bahrt to get back to running. She describes her comeback philosophy: "You don't come back better; the goal is to reach for the same level as before the injury," she states realistically. And she's scared of injuring herself again. She joins her Millrose teammates at speed workouts but is now at the back of the pack. "Sometimes when I'm running I feel like I am flying at an 8:30 pace. Then I look at my watch and see it was really a 9:30 pace," she laughs. "It's amazing how our mind can fool us into thinking we are flying, but I guess it means I am having fun and just happy to be running at all. Screw the pace—it's overrated!"

As for keeping her knee injury at bay, she will do what it takes to keep running until she can't. She runs every other day and swims and does Pilates on the other days. "I definitely won't throw in the towel . . . people deal with a lot worse. I keep telling myself, it's not my age, it's my knee!" As an artist (Bahrt is an award-winning children's knitwear designer), she relies on her running to bring clarity to her creativity. "It's those miles and miles that allow unfiltered creative thoughts to flow through," she states. "Nothing is more powerful than running to get you in the best shape—physically and mentally—and nothing is more terrifying than when that is taken away."

Bahrt and I end the interview reminiscing about high school days. We agree that the cross-country runners and soccer players were cooler than the football players. We saw each other once or twice during our college years but lost touch until I saw her running in Central Park one day and we rekindled our friendship. Amy is still cool and follows her own drumbeat.

When we meet, we talk about running and training and what our next race is. We gab about who is getting out of our age group—always a plus—and who is coming in—always a negative. And it still amazes us that our running lives started under the cover of darkness when we were teenagers, uncertain where it would take us but knowing that it would always be with us.

Gordon Bakoulis

DOB: February 14, 1961

Residence: Manhattan, New York

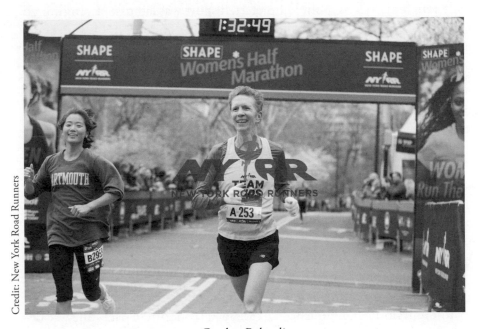

Gordon Bakoulis

"I can't imagine running not being in my life."
Gordon Bakoulis has an impressive running career that includes qualifying for the US Olympic marathon trials five times, competing as a finalist in the 1992 US Olympic 10,000-meter trials, and placing first in her age group at the 2001 New York City Marathon in 2:41:43 as

a forty-year-old. A former editor-in-chief of *Running Times* magazine, she just celebrated fifteen years with New York Road Runners (NYRR) as an editor and coach and, most importantly, as a respected co-worker. Bakoulis is gracious and unpretentious, and she's always giving back to the sport that has given her so much. She and her husband, Alan Ruben, are a formidable force on the racing circuit.

Bakoulis describes herself while growing up in Princeton, New Jersey as "a skinny geek." Her family was always active, and they instilled in her a love of being outdoors and being healthy. "We took a lot of family walks, did chores like cleaning the house and raking leaves," says Bakoulis. "I was always outdoors playing with the other kids, games like tag." Her father was a member of NYRR, and Bakoulis would occasionally join him on a run, but her preferred sport was lacrosse. Even though she loved the sport, she admits that she wasn't good at it. "I was totally uncoordinated. I loved to play but wasn't that great," she recalls. In her senior year of high school she switched to track and finally felt like she was good at something. Although her team was terrible, she won almost every race.

After high school she attended the University of Virginia. She looked into joining the track team, but after a talk with the coach, she changed her mind. "He made me realize that college track was a whole other level of running than in high school and it would take a lot of hard work and commitment," Bakoulis recalls. "I wanted to experience the full college life, which to me included pizza, beer, and staying out all night if I wanted to. So I chose to have a blast and I enjoyed my four years of college."

She ran one race in her freshman year, a ten-miler, and won without any training. In her senior year she ran a half marathon, again without training, and finished in 1:34, a 7:10-per-mile pace. She was beginning to realize that her natural talent for running extended to longer distances.

After graduating in 1983, Bakoulis moved to New York City and landed a job with *Ms.* magazine. That same year, she and her dad volunteered at the New York City Marathon. After they'd done their job of helping runners check in, they went to watch the finish. It was the year that Rod Dixon and Geoff Smith dueled for the win in the final stretch, and she was captivated by the thrill of it. She also enjoyed watching "the parade of humanity pass by and thought, I can do this!" She entered the lottery for the 1984 New York City Marathon, got in, and started training in July. She found a running partner who had finished a marathon, and she soaked up his knowledge. She did tempo runs and speed drills, kept a log, and learned how to hydrate on the run. As race day grew closer, she got super-excited. Back then it was still something of an anomaly for women to run marathons. Bakoulis didn't consider herself a real runner yet. "It wasn't part of my essence as it is now," she says.

She was well prepared on race day. "I had a healthy respect for what I was about to do," says Bakoulis, then twenty-three. "I knew this day would be different from anything I had ever done before." But race day was hot, 79 degrees Fahrenheit. She started with a friend, but by mile 10, Bakoulis picked up the pace and never looked back. She ran smart, taking in lots of fluids and backing off her pace when needed. She ran a consistent race and enjoyed herself along the way, taking in the sights of the five boroughs like a tourist. She finished in a respectable 3:40:03 and knew she was hooked.

Shortly after the marathon, she was recruited to run for an elite racing team. In 1987 she ran Grandma's Marathon in Duluth, Minnesota in 2:46 and felt like she'd found her calling. "I finally saw myself as a serious runner," says Bakoulis. That was more than thirty years ago. Since then she has represented the United States at the 1989 World Cup Marathon, the 1991 World Championships Marathon, the 1992 World Championships Half-Marathon, and the 1992 Beijing International Ekiden. She has PRs of 2:33:01 (marathon), 1:11:34 (half marathon), and 32:45 (10K), and she has twice finished among the top ten women in the New York City Marathon. In 2010, NYRR named her the 2000–09 Runner of the Decade. (But she won't tell you any of that. Instead, she'll ask you how your races are going.)

In 1996 she married Ruben, another fast runner, whom she met while training with the Central Park Track Club. They got engaged on a flight back from her 1996 Olympic Trials race. Their marriage was featured in the *New York Times* "Vows" column. They played tag-team with their running while raising three kids, trading who went out first and who stayed home with the children. Those years flew by.

At fifty-seven, Bakoulis is still a top contender but realizes she is slowing down a bit. She comments on her aging: "I don't feel young anymore! And due to that, I appreciate my running more every day than I ever did. I realize what a gift it is especially when I see friends who are going though injuries or are just in a decline. Or when I go to high school or college reunions and I see some of my peers. The effects of aging are more prevalent in people who don't exercise. That's why I consider running a gift that I want to preserve as long as I can, and why I take care of myself."

That means not doing super-hard workouts, taking more recovery time, and avoiding the track. She doesn't belong to a gym but will drop and do push-ups on the kitchen floor while cooking dinner. She's kept her mileage relatively high, running forty miles a week and up to sixty for marathon training. She runs seven days per week either on her own or while coaching, which she's done since 1985, and also rides her bike to work. In October of 2017, she ran her first marathon in three and a half years and was looking forward to a winning day. But as anyone who has run a marathon knows, it isn't as much about the training as the day of the race, and it was warm and raining. "I went out too fast and by mile 19 broke down to a nine-minute pace," she recalls. Despite her bad run she still placed first in her age group in 3:24. She doesn't believe in "revenge marathons" but will do another by the end of 2018.

Her favorite pastime when not running is walking all over Manhattan, and she's thrilled to be living in such a vibrant city. She does fun-runs with her husband and kids along the Hudson River Greenway or in Central Park. "We are so fortunate to be around parks," says Bakoulis.

On the work side of things, the four or five magazine issues that she edited per year are now down to one or two, so she is engaged in NYRR's digital and online presence. And she's taken to social media like a kid. Her Instagram account is active and full of terrific running shots from all over the city and wherever she visits. Her wide smile and red hair seem to vibrate off the screen with her enthusiasm and zest for life.

Bakoulis finds it a bit easier to accept slowing down because she came into the sport as a recreational runner before she became a competitive runner at the top. "Some elite runners have trouble continuing to run once they stop winning and setting records because they don't know what it's like to run for fun, to just enjoy running for pleasure," says Bakoulis. "It can get scary when you start setting up performance goals and tie your entire identity into that. I've been lucky to manage my identity as an elite runner along with my roles as a mother and wife, and in my career."

After nearly forty years of running, Bakoulis credits her ability to run seven days a week and race hard when she needs to with her passion for running and the healthy lifestyle it brings with it. She's known the pain and struggles it takes to be at the top of the heap, but she also loves running 5Ks with her twelve-year-old son and doesn't care when those slow results show up online. She's confident in her own skin, whether out in front or among the mid-packers. And as most aging runners come to realize, she's more apt to look at her age-graded percentile than any other measurement of her effort. She took first place age-graded at the New Balance Fifth Avenue Mile in September of 2017 at age fifty-six, finishing in 5:35, a 96.64 age-graded percentile. You can call her an outlier for that, but she's a gracious and humble one.

Summing up her running life, Bakoulis says, "I get as much as I give from the sport that I love so much. I plan to preserve this gift for as long as I can." Her advice to other senior runners is to enjoy it, respect it, and take time to look around and enjoy the view: "I've learned to appreciate every day that I'm able to go for a run. I remember how I felt when I played running games around my neighborhood as a kid—how it was a way to explore and engage and challenge myself, and how afterward I felt wonderful—strong, accomplished, full of energy yet calm. These days, running makes me feel the exact same way, and it can spark those feelings in anyone. I try to put those feelings first, and I try to create platforms for other runners to do the same. Because they won't be disappointed."

George Banker

DOB: December 16, 1949

Residence: Fort Washington, Maryland

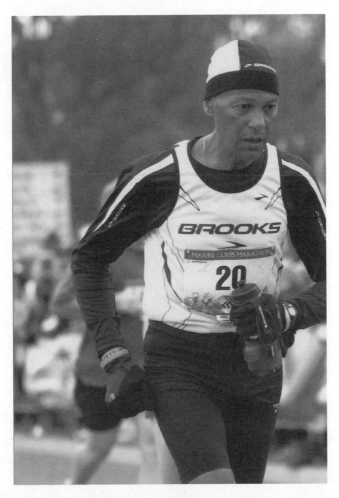

George Banker

"Determined, not deterred."

George Banker, a retired Technical Sergeant (TSgt.) in the US Air Force and former administrator with IBM, has run 110 marathons. He clocked his hundredth at his favorite marathon, the 2014 Marine Corps Marathon (MCM), which also was his thirty-first consecutive Marine Corps Marathon having only missed one since he started running them in 1983. He has also participated in seven fifty-mile races and was averaging fifty miles per week prior to his heart surgery in 2017. Nothing keeps Banker down. "If you want something bad enough, you will do whatever it takes to get it done," he says.

Banker came highly recommended to me as someone that I needed to include in my book and after reading about him, I knew why. Right off the bat I liked his old-school manner—he's never worn a heart rate monitor—and his passion for running. It oozes from him. He's a historian of the sport, a coach, and a writer, and he's involved in some level at most of the Washington, DC area's races, including the Army Ten-Miler, the Navy-Air Force Half Marathon, and the George Washington Parkway Classic. During our first interview I felt as if he was interviewing me, that I better ask the right questions. I think I passed the test. Banker doesn't like to waste time. He's a bundle of energy and a force to be reckoned with. He's tough and demanding but fair. This is how he describes his coaching style: "I will get inside your head; I want you to make a commitment. Take a look at your schedule. How much time do you have to devote? That's how much time you give. You need to get out of it what you want." What else would you expect from someone who spent most of his life in the military?

Banker's father was a Marine, as was his stepfather. He was born at Fort Monmouth in New Jersey and spent his childhood on bases, which shaped his life and how he looks at the world. "There is a bond that the military has that is very difficult to duplicate in civilian life," he said. "If I had to do it all again, I would choose that (military) life."

As a kid, he was always active. He played tennis and Little League baseball and was on a swim team. He walked most places and raced his brothers for fun. He also played football until he got tired of getting hit. As part of being a military kid, he learned discipline and structure. His stepfather would post a weekly work schedule of the chores Banker and his brother needed to do. "We knew exactly what chores had to be completed before we went out to play," he recalls. On Saturdays the job was to strip the wax off the floors with hot water and oven cleaner. Then they had to break the stove down and clean it with steel wool.

He joined the Air Force in 1969 and rose to the rank of a TSgt. ("I'm the guy who drove the fuel trucks onto the tarmac"). His major form of exercise was running to the package store for beer. He completed eight years of active duty from 1969 to 1977, which included service in Thailand. That was followed by twelve years in the DC Air National Guard based at Andrews Air Force Base, Maryland. While in the reserves he studied accounting at George Washington University, which led to a career at IBM for twenty-five years. During those years he and his wife Bernadette (they've been married for forty-seven years) raised three kids.

He picked up running in 1982 while working for IBM. Every summer, his office sponsored a one-mile run, which the branch director won every year. When they asked Banker, then thirty-two, to participate in it he thought he'd kick the butt of the "old gray-haired man." Well, he didn't win it, didn't even come close. He ran a twelve-minute mile and thought he'd die. "It was ugly," recalls Banker with a laugh. "I was looking for the rescue squad afterward and went home and poured myself a Chivas Regal and lit up my pipe."

He decided to become a better a runner and started consuming running magazines. He saw an advertisement for the 1982 Philadelphia Distance Run (half marathon) and felt that would be a good first race to try. His goal was to finish in two hours; he ran it in 1:59:00. "I thought I was tearing up that road so bad that they would need to resurface it after I got through running over it," he says laughing. "What a rush! Everything was clicking just right, and I felt that I had something." Banker is a talker and he can hold an audience with his stories and humor. He's fun to listen to.

After that half marathon, he was hooked. Seven months later he ran his first marathon, the Penn Relays Marathon in Philadelphia. He still has that T-shirt. His goal was an ambitious 3:30, but he finished in 4:24, making all the rookie mistakes. The cramps started at mile 16, and he willed himself to finish. He remembers it like a bad dream: "I called myself every name in the book and swore I would never do that again." But Banker is not a quitter.

He joined the Rock Creek Running Club and got serious about running. The training and camaraderie paid off and he ran his second marathon and first Marine Corps Marathon (MCM) four months later in 3:39. That's when he decided to embrace the running life and quit the Chivas Regal and the pipe. The following year he ran MCM in 3:09. At this point in our interview I asked him why he's drawn to running. His short answer is, "Because I like it." His longer answer: "Running gives me a sense of well-being. It has too many positive effects not to like it. Yes, there is a lot of hard work and time given up, but it is for the greater good the way I look at it. It forces you to get in tune with your body and mind. You learn to manage your time better. And let's not forget the people you meet and if you stay in the sport long enough, you'll see them again on a starting line."

After his first MCM, running took over his life when he wasn't at his desk at IBM. He was asked to be a scorer for local races and when he proved he was good at that, well-organized and efficient, he moved up to race director. He started writing a racing report for a local newspaper and was dubbed "the race reporter for the masses." He loved the stories of all the runners, not just the elites. "Everyone has a story," he says, "and I wanted to hear them, cry with them, and laugh with them." Through all this, he found the time to run six marathons each year with no injuries. "Everything just fell into place," he says. Even when he felt over his head, he never panicked or worried. "It was like changing a flat tire when the car is moving." As a race organizer, he was a hustler getting free pizzas delivered to a local evening race, repurposing trophies, and talking his way into getting free tech-fabric T-shirts for a new race.

By 1987 he was running 1:02 for ten miles at age thirty-five. He ran like a manic—but interestingly he credits running with keeping him balanced mentally and physically: "Running gives me that reason to keep going. It gives me an opportunity to help others and it's not always about speed and PRs. It's all about doing what makes your heart happy. Running helps me to stay focused and set goals and to go after them."

Banker also found that in running he pushed himself beyond his comfort zone and learned how to block out the pain. That allowed him to run his marathon PR of 3:04 set at the 1988 Houston-Tenneco Marathon. Running in old-school fashion, he drank only water on the course and wore his basic sports watch.

The years merged into one endless run for Banker. He worked countless hours both behind and in front of the racing scene around the DC area. His many roles included announcer, race director, troubleshooter, reporter, and scorer. He was an events jack-of-all-trades. "I'm an organized pack rat," he said. "When I die, there's going to be a U-Haul in the funeral procession, behind the hearse," he laughs.

And as the years flew by, before he knew it he was running his one-hundredth marathon—the MCM in 2014. It was a momentous occasion for him. His wife and kids were at the finish wearing T-shirts that read, "Team George." They presented him with a T-shirt of his own which read, "I did it!" That was followed by a celebratory cake and a big sign with his photo on it. "I still get chills thinking about that day," says Banker.

After his hundredth, he noticed that his times were getting slower and his breathing was labored and erratic. He knew something wasn't right but ignored it. He hadn't been to a doctor in twenty-six years, but after experiencing excruciating shoulder pain, he realized it was time to see one. In September of 2015, he saw a doctor at Walter Reed Hospital and was diagnosed with atrial fibrillation. He ran three more marathons with the new goal of making it to the finish before the cutoff time.

The following October, another visit to Walter Reed and more tests revealed a leaky heart valve, commonly known as mitral valve prolapse. Despite the news, a few weeks later he participated in his thirty-second MCM (playing number 103 overall). His wife glared at him. His doctor wasn't thrilled. But Banker was not going to stop his MCM streak.

Eventually, like a house of cards, his running came crashing down, as he could not ignore the pain and the required surgery he needed. The straw that broke the camel's back was having to DNF at his next race, a fifty-miler. In July of 2017 he underwent heart surgery to correct his mitral valve prolapse and irregular heartbeat, and what was supposed to be a four-hour surgery ended up taking seven hours due to hemorrhaging.

After the surgery, Banker was forced to rest for the remainder of the year. It drove him crazy not to run, but he remained focused and positive during his recovery. "I do not allow myself to sit back and say, why me? I thank God that I pulled through because I was almost lost. I had to be taken back into the operating room and my chest reopened. The operation was on a Monday and that Wednesday I was on my feet. I started back walking and using the stationary bike and elliptical two months later. I was letting my body tell me what I could do," reports Banker.

Now recovered, he doesn't waste time thinking about his past performances. "The beauty is that I know what I used to do but I do not know what I can do. The thrill is to try and find out. I have no desire to try and set a PR at any distance and then be in rehab for weeks," explains a subdued Banker. He weighs in on aging in general combined with his comeback after surgery. "It now takes more work to overcome the aging body as it's not as flexible. My age is now a factor in setting goals. Let me get real, I'm not training for the Olympics, so whatever I run is good in my book. Aging is a good thing. It gives us the experience we need to move forward in a positive direction and leads to the question, Why do I want to run faster and who cares? I set a record. Guess what? Two days later it's broken. I know what it takes to run a 3:30 marathon. The question is, what will it do for me? Do I really have the time to do the additional speedwork? Whew! I am getting tired just thinking about it. I can run a six-hour marathon and still say 'Oh baby, I did it!'"

Banker celebrated the 2018 New Year with a six-mile run, his longest distance since the surgery. His new goal is a ten-mile race in March and he will be very realistic about that goal. "I can't stop the aging process, and nor do I want to. I will continue to run for as long as I can, and my body will let me know when it's had enough. I know what I can and cannot do. I have the confidence that I can make the distance." His training includes a walk/run regimen, gradually cutting the walking down and increasing the runs and the pace. "I don't need a watch anymore to know I did my best because that's all I give," he says.

Banker is staying healthy, happy, and hungry for more adventures and races. His new motivator is not a PR but his health and heart. He gets up at 4:30 a.m. and is at the gym by 5:00. "Anything past five hours of sleep is unproductive time," he says. "I hit 110 marathons. How many more are left? How old is dirt?" Like many aging competitive runners, he looks forward to the next new age division because "everyone slows down at some point." At sixty-eight, he's had many thrilling life experiences. "God gave me the talent to be a journalist and a photographer and also the ability to run. It is through running that I have the opportunity to meet other people who have enriched my life." His biggest achievement—besides marrying the perfect woman—is capturing his thirty years of history with the MCM in a book he wrote in 2007, *The Marine Corps Marathon: A Running Tradition,* which he describes as a labor of love.

Banker is still going to run like a crazy man, but with less intensity. He's gone thirty years without a drop of alcohol and just gave up coffee. He stopped eating meat ten years ago and doesn't miss it. When faced with a decision, he asks himself, "How bad do you want this?" For Banker, the answer is always "I want it all!"

Kathy Bergen

DOB: December 24, 1939

Residence: La Cañada Flintridge, California

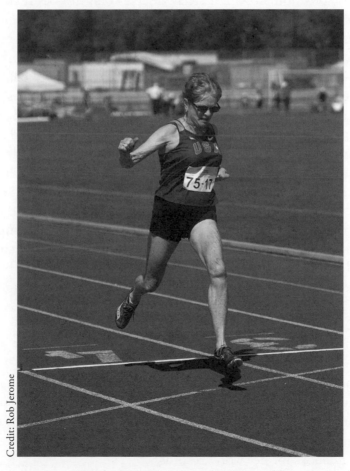

Kathy Bergen winning the 100m gold

"We're all nuts!"

In 2015, seventy-five-year-old Kathy Bergen ran 14.76 in the 100 meter-dash, becoming the oldest woman to run under fifteen seconds. In 2017 she set an American record at the Albuquerque Masters Indoor Championships in the 200-meter dash. She also competed in the high jump and 60-meter dash. She is considered one of four of the best women in the history of masters sprinting in US history. Bergen didn't start competing until she was fifty-four when her husband entered her into a masters' championship. When she asked him what event she would do without any training or preferred sport he said, "Just run. Anyone can run." And run she did, and high jump and throw the javelin and set world records. A spry woman with a steely reserve, Bergen doesn't mind the hard work she puts into her training because as she states, "I love to win!"

Kathy Bergen was born on Christmas Eve. She never got a real party as a child, so later in life she unofficially changed her birthday to July 24 so she could have a pool party. That date change could have been an early omen that when Bergen wants something, she goes after it, whether it be a birthday party or a world record. Raised in the Bay Ridge section of Brooklyn, New York, she was an only child but had a lot of male cousins. She has fond memories of playing with them. "The street was our playground," she recalls. "We played stickball, rode our bikes, and roller-skated. I did whatever the boys did." She had no idea that she was fast, coordinated, or competitive. She just kept up with the boys, sometimes beating them. Like many women who became competitive late in life, she wonders what she could have been capable of if allowed. "I would so love to know what I could have done as a teenager, but back then, there weren't many outlets for women's sports," says Bergen. She refers to the lack of athletics for women in the 1950s as a great disappointment in her life.

In high school she played basketball, but girls were only allowed to play half-court with three on defense and three on offense. "Females were considered delicate flowers back then," she laughs. "I was a terrible shot." At Marymount Manhattan College she majored in economics, which she remembers as so boring and wishes she had been a history major. Interesting that she would have selected history as she is now in the history books for her world records.

She worked for a while at General Motors in the Treasurer's Office, a job she considered very boring. In 1963 at age twenty-three, she married and had three kids before moving to California with her husband, Bert. She took up tennis and fell in love with the sport. There's a trend here that Bergen does not like to sit still. They lived in California from 1972 to 1977 until her husband was transferred to Pleasantville, New York. She continued playing tennis but missed the California weather. Bert was transferred back to California in 1984 and she vowed she would never leave again. "I love being a New Yorker and will never forget my Brooklyn roots, but I love the California life-style," states Bergen. After getting to know Bergen I can't imagine this twirling dervish of a women sitting at a bank job, or sitting for any length of time at anything.

In 1994, while raising her five kids and playing competitive tennis, Bert spotted an AARP article about the Senior Olympic Games at nearby Occidental College. He had high-jumped in high school and decided to go to the games and see what it was all about. He asked Kathy if she wanted to come along and she wondered what sport she would do. He replied, "Try running. Everyone can run." So Kathy, at the age of fifty-four, entered her first track meet and fell in love with it. She ran the 50- and 100-meter and won both. She was on a high. When she and Bert lived in New York they attended the Millrose Games in Madison Square Garden and loved seeing all the track-and-field events. Now, she was competing in one and had to pinch herself she felt so lucky. That first meet will always hold a special place in her heart for introducing her to a new world.

While at the meet they found a copy of *National Masters News*. Today it's an online publication but back then it was a published newspaper. They were both shocked and happy to find that there was a whole world of masters' track-and-field meets just waiting for them to sign up for. They started attending all the local meets and had a ball. Shortly after, their youngest son graduated high school, so Kathy had even more time to train. She ran around a track a few days a week, nothing too strenuous. She and Bert look back at that time with fond memories of attending track meets and meeting a whole new circle of friends. Bert stuck with his high jump and Kathy ventured out, exploring all sorts of sports. She was like a kid in a candy shop. The high jump, the javelin, the discus, shot put, and the sprint distances—she tried them all. "It was so much fun and I met great people," she states. "I met people as nutty as I was about sports!" The other thing she loved about being around athletes at the meets is that no one talks about their illnesses. "No one says, oh my blood pressure is high, or I'm on this and that medication," she states. "We talk about how our training is going and complain about a few nagging running aches and pains and what meet we are going to next."

She remembers buying her first pair of track spikes and gear. "I bought purple shorts and a matching singlet," she recalls. "The kids laughed like crazy when they saw me in my 'official' track outfit." At the meets she had to get used to running in mixed age groups. There weren't many women in her age group running track so they ran in mixed ages from fifty up, or seventy and up. "Our ages are written on the bib so we do know where we are positioned," explains Bergen. "And at the end, we are only judged in our specific age groups."

Her first championship event was in 1996 at Reno. She entered the 60-meter Indoor and set an age-group American record. For Bergen, it's always win or lose. There is no middle ground. Her reaction at breaking the record was typical Bergen: "Holy cow! I broke it!" She didn't end there. She went on to try out the high jump. She watched the other high jumpers practice and decided to give it a try. "The high jumpers were so supportive and taught me about the two styles of jumping, the straddle approach and the Fosbury Flop, named after Dick Fosbury who won gold at the 1968 Olympics by going over the bar backwards." A few months later at the 1996 Outdoor Nationals she set an American age-group record in the high jump with the Flop.

She came close to not competing in the high jump at all, lovingly threatened with divorce from a concerned husband. According to an article on Ken Stone's website, masterstrack.com, Bergen suffered a serious injury while training for the high jump: "It was 1996. She was laid up for eight months after her back went out and Kathy's husband, Bert, didn't want to see her hurt again. To drive the point home, Bert told her that if she ever high jumped again, he would divorce her. Two years later, in better health, Bert relented and Kathy was back trying the flop. She has since dominated the high jump in her age group, and in 2006 soared to indoor and outdoor world records." In that same article on Bergen, she says she's not concerned about ever having to take a doping test for additives to make her even faster. "They can test me if they want," she said. "All they'll find is vodka and wine."

In her sixties, Bergen set more American records in the 60-64 age division. She concentrated in the 60-meter event, but at the big national meets she competes in the 200. When she hit sixty-eight, she noticed a decline in her speed and felt she was at a standstill, "spinning my wheels and going nowhere." Turning seventy, she read an article in the *National Masters News* about Eric Dixon, an online accredited track coach. She hired him, and after hearing her workout routine told her she was doing it all wrong. "I was doing all sorts of things every week like some track workouts, some tennis, high-jump practice, and weight strengthening. I was all over the place," says Bergen. He put her on a regime of thee days a week at the track with specific workouts, then two days a week at the gym doing weight strengthening with free weights and two complete rest-and-recovery days. She followed the schedule religiously, except for the tennis games she snuck in without reporting it. "His schedule built in recovery time which I rarely took and it gave me more endurance and energy at the meets," stated Bergen.

The partnership worked out well as Bergen went on to set fifteen World Age-Group Records in the 60-, 100-, and 200-meter dash and high jump both indoors and outdoors. "I worked really hard to achieve those goals, but I love it," says Bergen. "I love being physically fit and pushing myself to be the best I can be." Bergen talks about taking up sports late in life and how it opened up a new world for her. "I'm not trying to be young," she states up front. "But I'm not the type to sit on a couch and knit. That's not me. I've loved being active since I was a kid and the masters' games gave me the opportunity to finally be the athlete I always knew I could be."

She attends as many meets as she can, some for social reasons more than the competitive challenge. She saves her record attempts for the masters' track-and-field series and laments the fact that there aren't many women competing in her age division. She looks forward to the world meets where the European women have a deeper field. "They spur me on to compete harder," she states. She gets upset at open meets where she is the oldest woman competing against others at least ten years older, and although she holds her own, she doesn't get the credit for being the oldest. "The announcer just says, 'And last is Kathy Bergen' when the announcer should say, 'And last, at age seventy-eight, is Kathy Bergen,'" she states. "I think I deserve that." She does indeed.

When she doesn't win, she has learned to be philosophical instead of getting angry. "I've realized it's self-defeating to get angry if I don't win," says Bergen. "I used to do that but now I'll review a disappointing race with my coach and analyze where I could have done better and get back to work." But that doesn't happen often. In February 2018, she ran in a 200-meter exhibition at the Indoor National Championships in Albuquerque and won. Four of the women were in their sixties; Bergen was seventy-nine.

Humble, she feels some of the records she set are due to the fact that there is no competition in her age group and the old records are soft. Bergen doesn't want to just win, she wants to win with a fight and earn it. Like the time she crushed the W75 world record in the 100 meter at the 2015 Mount Sac Relays. As she states, "I'm making up for lost time!" She looks fifty, acts forty, and has a beautiful stride as she approaches the high jump, clearing the bar with practiced finesse. In her many interviews she is well-spoken, spunky, and full of life. She looks stylish and casual even in her track gear. If she weren't a world-class athlete she'd be a shoe-in for president of the PTA.

To Bergen, there is a mind-body correlation between being physically and mentally active. She attends meets as much for the competition as the social engagement. "I can't think of anything I'd rather do than be outdoors on a sunny day sitting around the track with my husband and friends all sweaty with sunblock, discussing our events. Bert and I are so lucky to be able to do this together and we both love it," says Bergen. A role model to her kids, she and Bert taught their children, and now grandchildren, to appreciate all sports and to give it their best. When she and Bert were raising their five kids they had a pool in the backyard so learning to swim was imperative. All of her kids went on to be collegiate swimmers. Bergen dabbled with competitive swimming for a period, even entering two meets with her kids. It didn't appeal to her but for those meets she entered she did well. It seems Bergen does everything well that she attempts.

Her goal when she turns eighty in two years is to keep breaking records. "I'm going after the WR 80 in the high jump and 100 and 200 meters," she states. She'll continue to experiment with other events "just because it's so much fun." She'll maintain her busy schedule of eight to ten events on the national circuit and if her endurance and hard work keeps up, she'll achieve her goals, and more. In order to do that, she needs to stay injury-free. Over the last twenty-four years she has pulled every muscle and tendon possible. Currently she is dealing with runner's knee and tennis elbow. She has a great physical therapist she's been seeing for twenty years who knows every nook and cranny in her body. She knows how important it is for athletes, especially older athletes, to remain injury free. "As you age it takes longer to recover. You cannot ignore injuries and compete when something hurts," states Bergen.

There are numerous ways to describe Bergen: plucky, fun-loving, spirited, and competitive come to mind. She was fortunate to find an outlet for sports late in life and has not missed a day loving the world she entered. She is a poster child for the benefits of staying active and attending senior games at all levels. Kathy and Bert Bergen are living the dream of positive aging and making it look easy. That's a lesson to adhere to every day: "As long as God gives me good health I'll keep doing what I do because I love it," she says.

Witold Bialokur

DOB: January 17, 1935

Residence: Queens, New York

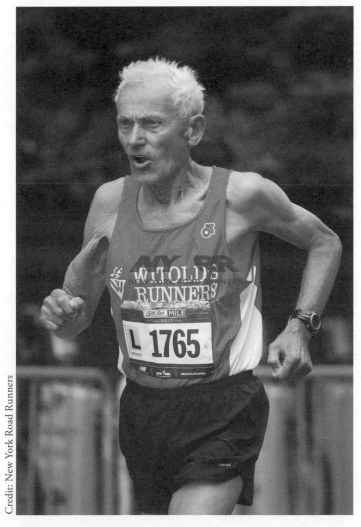

Witold Bialokur at the 5th Avenue Mile in 2017

Graceful Ageing and a Waltz.

Witold Bialokur is a living legend. Ask any runner in the tri-state area about him and they nod their heads and acknowledge his times and his winning appeal. In September of 2017 at age eighty-two, he ran the New York Fifth Avenue Mile in 7:04. Two weeks later he ran a ten-miler at a 9:06 pace. Bialokur follows a strict training discipline based on legendary distance runner Emil Zatopek's methods. Just ask any of the members of Witold's Runners, a club he founded in 1983 and still coaches. He does not take well to excuses and never asks anything of his members that he cannot do himself.

Bialokur is a welcome fixture at races. An elegant gentleman who opens doors for ladies and has been seen to bend and kiss the hand of a former elite runner in his age group, he is suave and handsome as a Hollywood star. He and Urszula, his wife of fifty years, are ballroom dance instructors, usually booked on cruises to teach the waltz, mambo, and tango. Don't be fooled by his elegance and piercing blue eyes. Underneath that old-world charm is a man with a killer instinct, a skill he crafted to survive as a youth in war-torn Poland.

Although I knew of Bialokur's running acclaim and had met him at NYRR club nights back in the 1990s, when the event was black tie, he was always a man of mystery to me. Tall, erect, with a swath of silver hair, everyone paid tribute to him. I knew I wanted to interview him for this book and searched him out. I had to go through a few layers of protection before I reached him. He has a loyal following of young friends and running buddies who protect his privacy and vet journalists looking for an interview. He agreed to meet me, and we finally sat down on a rainy afternoon in November to talk.

Bialokur was born in Poland at the outbreak of World War II. He was just three years old when Germany invaded Poland. His father, a Polish military officer, was sent to prison in Siberia and he never saw him again. Two weeks later, Russia invaded eastern Poland and fighting broke out along every border. His young mother was desperate to survive with her three kids and moved to the Russian border, now the Ukraine, finding refuge in a straw hut. Battles raged around them day and night. During cease-fires, Bialokur and his brothers would go out and search for food, sometimes dodging bullets. "I grew up in interesting times," he tells me as he sips hot tea across from me at a café in Manhattan. "We stole apples from orchards, anything to survive. Sometimes we hid in the bomb craters when the fighting started up again. This is where I learned to run fast," he adds.

After the war, his family moved to Krakow. He went to school to study engineering and ran with a government-sponsored running club, clocking a 4:15 mile. Living under Soviet Russian rule, he also had to serve in the Soviet Army. When they realized what a good runner he was they "asked him" to coach the team. He found that he loved coaching. He used training techniques based on Emil Zatopek's with great results. One of his runners competed in the 1968 Olympics. Despite his success with running, he hated living under Communist rule. In 1970, by then married to Urszula, he planned an escape that no one, not even his mother, knew about.

He had saved up to buy a two-cylinder car, which he describes as a Soviet-era plastic body car. One night during Christmas vacation he told his mother that he and Urszula were going on a vacation. As he tells me the story, Bialokur's eyes well up. "My mother looked at me and said, 'No one goes on vacation during Christmas. I doubt I will ever see you again. Go and do what you must.'" Before departing, he took one last run with his club and silently said goodbye to them as well. "They could feel it, they knew I was escaping and wished me well with silence," he adds.

The couple traveled to Vienna, stayed for three years, then moved on to Paris, and finally New York. He was thirty-eight and arrived with one daughter, Monique. His son, Michael, was born in New York in 1980. During those past ten years, he never ran. When he arrived in Queens and went for a walk in Flushing Meadows Corona Park, he saw people jogging. He recalls his reaction to seeing this new phenomenon: "I scratched my head in wonder. Why were they running so slowly? What was this activity? If they were running, why weren't they lined up in fashion like in cross-country or a track meet?" Bewildered, he didn't join the joggers. Instead, he joined a soccer team to keep in shape.

Settled in Queens with two kids, Bialokur got a job working for an engineering firm at the World Trade Towers. The company put out a newsletter and in 1983 advertised for runners who could break five hours in a marathon to form a company team. He signed up even though he hadn't run in ten years, confident of his abilities. He ran the New York City Marathon in 1984 in 3:54 at age forty-nine. He hated the experience. That marathon went down in NYRR history as the "the disaster of 1984," due to the oppressive weather. One runner died and dozens more were treated at area hospitals for heat-related conditions. The humidity ranged from 96 percent early in the day to 65 percent in the afternoon. It was downright torturous, but Bialokur finished.

After picking up running again, Bialokur became a regular at NYRR races. The younger runners kept up with him and took a liking to him. "They realized I knew what I was doing and they started to ask me to coach them," says Bialokur. That was the beginning of the club he started in 1983, Witold's Runners. There's a waiting list for new members and they have to pass the six-minute-mile test before joining. The group meets three times a week in Forest Park, Queens and Bialokur puts them through grueling workouts, time-tested from his days of coaching in the Soviet Union. He believes the best workouts are when you bring the body to total exhaustion—and then do more.

He doesn't ask his teammates to do anything he can't. In fact, he is probably harder on himself than anyone. And his race records are proof that Bialokur is at the top of his game. At fifty and fifty-one, Bialokur ran 4:40s for the mile. At sixty-two, he ran 5:14, defeating Canadian Earl Fee, who has set numerous world masters track records. Bialokur's 2015 mile time bettered the American age eighty-to-eighty-four mile record by almost ten seconds. In 2015, USA Track & Field named him the nation's top male performer in the eighty-to-eighty-four age-group. His team captain, Alan Novie, has nothing but praise for Bialokur: "When we see him approaching us for practice, it is with both great anticipation and a bit of dread! What will he have in store for us this weekend? How many drills with he put us through in the woods? How many loops on the horse trail will we have to run," says Novie, with all due respect. "I mention this because whatever we do and however difficult it is, Witold does it with us so we can't back down or not keep up because at eighty-three he just keeps going."

His strenuous training takes its toll on Bialokur and he admits to many injuries. "Lots of them," he laughs. "I try to ignore them but they always remind me they are still there." In his fifties, he dealt with chronic knee issues that kept him from competing at his prime for four years. He describes how he dealt with the injury: "I went to a fancy New York City doctor who told me I needed surgery. No way was I going to do that. So I went to a doctor in Poland I knew and respected and he sent me to a natural healing center with all sorts of homeopathic remedies and it worked. Six months later I was back in form." He visits the center once a year to soak in the sulfur baths and regenerate his tired muscles. "It stinks, but it is worth it," he adds.

He recalls his sixties as a great time for him. He set a goal to break six minutes at the Fifth Avenue Mile and accomplished it with time to spare in 5:12. He tells me how he reached his goal: "There were five of us at the start. I stay behind, keeping a nice pace. One guy drops out early. I start to pick up my pace and with 200 meters to go I see the finish line and start ripping it like a bullet. Sometimes you just have to let it all out and go for broke."

His seventies were another good decade. He retired from work and concentrated solely on his running and dancing. He kept a 7:30 pace for the half marathon and a 6:10 for the mile. Now in his eightieth decade, he is dealing with his loss of speed—although he ran the Fifth Avenue Mile in exactly 7:00 at age eighty—and a loss of running companions. He says he needs more recovery time, more sleep and tries to avoid injuries by listening to his body more. "I look at my competition at races and sometimes I am just competing with myself," he says. His strongest competitor is George Hirsch. They have a friendly respect for each other and Hirsch knows that when he sees Bialokur at the start, he is more than likely going to take second place.

Bialokur's goal now is to beat his time from the previous year, which he did at eighty-two. That year his mile time was 7:04, beating his previous year's time by a second. "At my age, seconds count a lot," he laughs. He's at peace with himself and can accept a slower time without causing a fuss. At eighty-three, he runs five days a week with a long run of ten miles on the weekends. He spends time with his twin grandchildren and dances three or four times a week. "Dancing is my cross-training," he adds. "That is where I get my balance, my flexibility, and elegance of movement. It is the perfect complement to running." He and Urszula are still doing dance instruction on cruises seven times a year. Sitting across from me at the café he mimics a few tango moves which draw applause from a few customers sitting nearby.

Bialokur is a modern Renaissance man. His life is full. He dances, paints, reads the classics, and listens to music. He doesn't take any medications. And he still climbs on the roof to fix leaks.

He describes his perfect day: "Go for a run, dance with my wife, have dinner out and end the day with a cognac." He tells me it is important in life to look at everything with a positive view. "I feel like I have wasted the day if I don't do something positive," he adds. At eighty-three, he feels like a very lucky man to have such a full life. But he also realizes that ageing has it side effects, like being invisible to the general population. "I look in the mirror in the morning when I am shaving or combing my hair and see a very distinguished and youthful person. Then I walk outside and no one sees me. I become invisible due to my age."

But anyone who knows Witold Bialokur knows he is anything but invisible. He has resisted the stereotypes of aging by living a healthy, active lifestyle. He has a lust for life that age will not diminish.

Karen Bowler

DOB: October 22, 1949

Residence: Cumbria, England, and Clermont, Florida

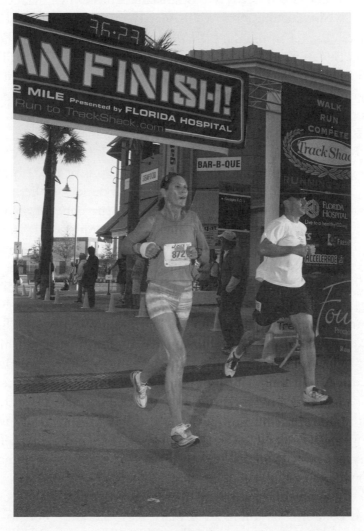

Karen Bowler

"Remember to smile when you run."

You definitely want Karen Bowler as your neighbor or a running partner. She would keep you on pace, keep you laughing, and at the end make you a nice cup of tea. How could you not want to run with someone who won the 1990 Hep Set Pyramid Marathon in Giza and posed with a photo of Fred Lebow wearing a pharaoh's costume? The local press called her "The Queen of the Nile." That story alone would keep you running and laughing for miles. Although not a household name in the United States, Bowler was a top distance runner in England during the 1980s. She was the 1985 Welsh Marathon champion and the 1987 World Veteran's champion in the 10K and 25K. She still enjoys her daily runs but gets more enjoyment from coaching runners and triathletes.

Bowler was born in Wales. As a little girl she ran everywhere. "I was very sporty and had a go at most sports," says Bowler in her proper British accent. She was fast and showed promise, so her parents sent her to a sports camp when was twelve. However, as a female she was restricted to the 800-meter event. That didn't sit right with her and she ended up running on the boys' teams. "After they made fun of me, I beat them all," she recalls. After that camp, there were no outlets for her to run so she pretty much stopped running. In school she concentrated in art, moving to London at eighteen, where she met her husband, Tim.

When she was thirty-two, married with children, she and Tim moved to the countryside where they bought a sixteenth-century farmhouse. Her husband joined a rugby team and ran a three-mile loop through town to stay in shape. Meanwhile, Bowler was busy rehabbing the house and taking care of the kids. One day, frustrated with the renovation and jealous of her husband's runs, she decided to join him. He looked a bit hesitant and told her not to get lost, as he would probably be faster. She laced up her green Dunlop tennis sneakers and took off. "To his surprise, I beat him back home," laughs Bowler. The next weekend she ran ten miles without breaking a sweat. She fell in love with running and the freedom she felt when running through the English countryside. She ran through the snow in winter and the blooms in the meadow in the spring.

A few months later, feeling like she had no limits, she decided to run the London Marathon. In January of 1982, she stood in line in the snow outside the local post office to mail her entry. While on the queue, she read about another marathon, the Seven Sisters Marathon, which courses over Sussex Downs. She ran that as her first marathon in February 1983 in a time of 5:17. Two months later she ran the London Marathon in a time of 3:47. At the time, it was the largest marathon in the world with a field of 15,116 participants.

After her mediocre finish time, Bowler decided she needed to train and take her running to a new level. But she had no one to train with, so she started her own running club, The Hailsham Harriers, for support. "I was tired of running in the streets alone and with no plan," she explains. The training and support paid off and the following year she qualified for the elite start at the 1984 London Marathon, finishing in 3:12. Two years later she won the 1986 Harrow Marathon in 3:01. She went from a non-runner to an elite in the span of three years, running eleven marathons and other distances during that time. Asking Bowler for her race times is an issue, as she never wrote anything down, saying, "It was so long ago." When I ask her how many marathons she's run, she says hundreds and then laughs. "I can't remember!" Thank goodness Tim keeps all the records.

During this time in her running career, she was busy raising kids. Her biggest challenge was keeping her running a secret from her parents. They did not approve. If they were at her house, she'd make up a story such as having to go food shopping. She'd change into her running clothes is a public bathroom, get in her run, then change out of her clothes in the public bathroom, do the food shopping, and go home to prepare dinner. When they asked why it took so long she'd make up an answer: "Oh, the shops were crowded and the queues were so long."

Speaking with Bowler on the phone is like having her sitting next to me. She hops from one topic to another and jumps out with stories from one marathon to the next. It's hard to keep track, but she is so much fun that I just try and keep up. When she mentions running the 1989 New York City Marathon with the elite field, I need to stop her for more details. "Oh dear," she says in her lovely English accent. "That was a disaster." The 1989 New York City Marathon was freezing, according to the then forty-year-old Bowler. The marathon website states that it was in the low fifties, but she remembers it as very cold. She stood at the elite start in her Union Jack shorts ready to give it her all, but between her jetlag and the weather, she ran a disappointing 3:04:59, a 7:03 pace.

Probably the craziest race Bowler ever did, which is a hint to just how plucky she can be, is the aforementioned 1990 Cairo Hep Set

Pyramids Marathon. Tim was working in Cairo for a computer systems company and the day before he was to fly home he saw an advertisement in the local paper for the marathon. He had kept up his running in the heat and difficult terrain in Cairo so he felt he was up for it and thought it would be far more fun if Bowler was by his side. He placed a call to her back in London. The marathon was the following day. At first Bowler thought he was crazy, but she caught a flight to Cairo and arrived at midnight. Eight hours later they were at the start line along with forty-six other runners. The course went by the Sphinx and pyramids, but the runners were chased by packs of wild dogs and ran through dirty canal water. Donkeys were crossing in front of them, carrying pallets of dung. Sometimes there's a water stop, sometimes not. They stuck together for the first half until Bowler took off, leaving him literally in the dust. By the time he finished, Bowler was being interviewed by the press as the first—and only—female finisher in a time of 3:14.

Bowler continued running marathons and races at other distances, training fifty or more miles a week. When friends or new runners asked her for help, she was happy to oblige as she was already an experienced coach with the Hailsham Harriers. In fact, she got more out of helping others than running races herself. In 1995, her husband was transferred to Houston, so the family packed up and moved to Texas. She continued racing and competing until she met Sabra Harvey. They were friendly rivals in the same age-group. Bowler saw the raw talent hidden in Harvey and offered to coach her. "Instead of competing against her I decided to help her win," laughs Bowler. Their friendship and coaching still remain strong today. In late 2018 she'll accompany Harvey to the World Masters Track and Field Championships in Malaga, Spain.

That's at the point that Bowler started coaching. At sixty-two, her running was slowing down due to Lyme disease from a tick bite. Her stamina took a hit due to the illness. When asked how she felt about leaving competitive running, she doesn't miss a beat: "You never stop competing in your head, just on your feet. I could give it up because I had such a full life beyond the running," says Bowler philosophically. "I feel very blessed to have such a positive life that I can share with others. I've been told that I have saved lives from clients who were obese and turned into athletes. I still can feel the hug I received from a client with Parkinson's disease who I trained to race a 5K and who went on to compete in an Ironman. I can see the physical changes in these people and the wonderful achievements made by them."

Many of her running clients are in the masters' category; a group she feels doesn't get the attention it deserves. According to Bowler, "Most experts come to the conclusion that competitive senior athletes rely on good genes, a keen interest in sport, and a lot of good luck." Bowler doesn't buy into that theory. She has coached many seniors who set new PRs into their seventies. She feels older people make the best students because they have a strong desire to succeed and a shorter amount of time to get there. "They bring their multi-faceted life experiences to the table and that is priceless," says Bowler. She cites the Olympic gold medalist Fanny Blankers-Koen as a role model for seniors and gives them homework assignments to read about her. I admit I had never heard of Blankers-Koen and had to Google her. She is extraordinary. She was a Dutch housewife who emulated Jesse Owens and competed in the 1936 Berlin Olympics, where she got a coveted autograph from him. She finished a disappointing fifth in the women's 4x100-meter relay but kept training and went on to win four gold medals in track and field at the 1948 London Olympics at the age of thirty.

At her first meeting with a new client, Bowler asks about goals. "They need to understand that goals should be realistic, so sometimes we need to reset a goal to make it achievable," she says. The second step in her coaching is an evaluation of balance and flexibility to determine what level of training they are suited for, whether it's a beginner who has to build core strength and balance or an experienced runner who needs to tweak a few things. "I need to determine where their strength lies and what needs to be adjusted, built, or changed, adds Bowler. "It's like building a pyramid. You need to have a strong foundation or there is a risk of injury and the pyramid topples." Finally, she asks about diet. She insists on a healthy diet as the second most important base of the pyramid.

Bowler also gets into the heads of her clients. She believes that the mind has to be exercised as much as the body, especially as we age. Part of this mindset is being engaged in society. You'll never catch Bowler living in a gated community or a senior residential complex. "We need to be among all ages, all abilities, and all backgrounds to stay alert and aware of our world," she says firmly. This past Halloween at age sixty-eight, she dressed up as a witch and ran in a local 5K.

Part of her coaching also deals with helping competitive athletes let go of past performances, which can be difficult for some. "You can't live on past performances," she says. "I try to get them to see that there are different levels of achievement and they can still achieve many goals." Sometimes it's really a matter of confidence. When an athlete stops winning, they can lose confidence and give up altogether. She encourages them to look for the passion they had when they first started running and brew it back up again. Then she deals out the tough love part and tells them no one is invincible so get over yourself.

Some of her favorite clients are the older ones who have never run before but want to get in shape, lose weight, or because their doctor advised it. She starts with a walking program on a field, pointing out the scenery, chats away with them and gets to go a little further every time they meet. Then she introduces a little jogging, interspersed with the walking. "I let them increase the jogging and distance at their leisure," says Bowler. "They need to build the confidence at one level before moving to the next." She keeps it nice and simple and social. The key is not to have them get injured. She preaches to all her aged fifty and above clients that they need to be flexible and have a strong core not only for running but also for daily life activities. She truly believes that exercise and aging well go hand in hand.

Other aspects of her coaching include cross training. She loves aqua jogging and recently has taken up spin classes along with strength training. "At our age we can't run hard every day," she explains. "Sometimes I'll just go out for a two-mile run and call it a day." Other days she'll run for thirty minutes followed by a ten-miler on the weekend. She also does mental prep work with her clients and teaches them to listen to their bodies. Many coaches use this term, but Bowler actually teaches what it means. She starts at the top of the head and works her way down, all the while asking, "How does this feel today?" She also believes in warming the muscles before exercising then stretching and icing afterward. She doesn't believe in static stretching before running but does active stretching such as high knees, butt kicks, and lunges. Says Bowler, "You want to warm up the muscles and relax them to avoid injuries. Run relaxed, not tense." Bowler practices what she preaches. After a long run she'll draw an ice bath, brew a cup of tea, and sit in the bath fully clothed while sipping her hot tea.

None of her coaching has been for monetary reasons. She strongly believes that coaching should be rewarded by results and not by a paycheck as it can alter the motivation for putting in the hard work and most importantly the mentoring aspect of coaching. "My passion for the sport and passing that on to others is its own reward," says Bowler. "All I ask is a friendly note when they have reached their goals." She treasures those notes that far exceed any monetary payment.

Bowler's biggest belief for maintaining a long, healthy life, is to smile every day. According to Bowler, "It's important to smile as it relaxes the face and makes everyone feel good. I spend a lot of time smiling. My life has been a wonderful journey and the best part is that it isn't over yet."

Michael Brooks

DOB: November 17, 1945

Residence: Lewiston, Maine

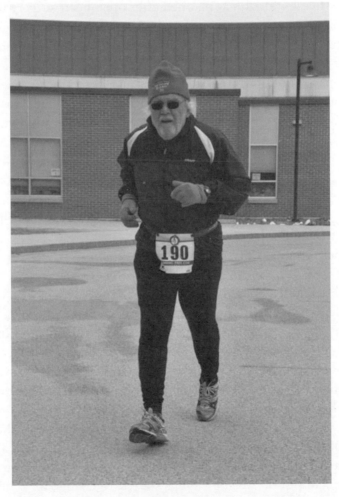

Michael Brooks

"Just call me Old Slow Mike."

When I interviewed Mike, he had just finished running seven marathons in seven days at age seventy. His next milestone was running his five-hundredth marathon, but first, he had to have open-heart surgery. When he told his doctors he was going to run a marathon within three months of his surgery they told him he was crazy. But never bet against Mike. Three years ago his doctors warned him about his heart and said he could drop dead at any point. That was over two hundred races ago. He ran his five-hundredth marathon as planned on October 2 in Portland, Maine. I caught up with him by phone afterward and he told me, "I did my five-hundredth as planned after open heart surgery to replace my aortic valve. Then back in the hospital for another week due to infection. Feeling much better now but very slow running. Plan on running just as many races in future." His optimism has no bounds.

Brooks started running at fifty and averages seventy races a year. He has served on the board of the 50 States Marathon Club as an investigator of runner fraud and is a member of the Mega Marathon List, where entry is a minimum of three hundred marathons. But Mike was not always a runner. In fact, if you had asked forty-nine-year-old Mike if he could see into the future and recognize the man who ran five hundred marathons, he'd die laughing interspersed with a coughing fit from smoking two packs of cigarettes a day and his oversized belly would shake with laughter.

Brooks grew up in Sommerville, Massachusetts, part of an Irish-Catholic family. It was a tough place with lots of gangs back then. He hated school, barely making it through. He started smoking at age ten, picking up butts off the streets. He never ran, "except when the cops were chasing us." After high school he worked at a shipyard in Boston but then gravitated up to Maine. While there, he read an advertisement for a firefighter and took the exam. "Back then, the exam was easy," recalls Brooks. "The recruiter held up two fingers and asked me how many I saw. When I said two, he told me I passed the test."

He stayed for thirty-three years, working his way up to chief, retiring in 2001. In 1983, he started running to help him through a divorce, but it was a short-lived dip that only lasted two years. He started smoking again and put on weight. Things started to change for the better in 1992 when he signed up for a 150-mile bike ride fundraiser for multiple sclerosis to help out a fellow firefighter whose wife was diagnosed with the disease. After that, he made a vow on Christmas morning 1994 to run to work every morning, a 6.2-mile run. It wasn't easy. At the time, he was forty-nine years old, weighed 235 pounds, and smoked. "I had to walk/run for the first few days until I could run the entire way," says Brooks.

His first race was a 5K. To train, he joined the Lewiston Running Club. After the race, he told the race director that he wanted to qualify for Boston. In October, a few months later, he ran his first marathon with the goal of qualifying and did so in 3:38. But that wasn't enough. A month later he ran the New York City Marathon and signed up for the January Fat Ass Marathon in Topsfield, Massachusetts, but he had to drop out due to an injury. He ran Boston in 1996.

I was beginning to see a trend in Brook's running, kind of a take-no-prisoners approach. "My doctor thinks I'm obsessive-compulsive," laughs Brooks. I think the doctor's right. After Boston, Brooks did his first 50-miler, followed by a 100-miler, and the 135-mile Badwater course in California's Death Valley in 2004. He ran 491 miles in a ten-day race. He's done a marathon or ultra in every state five times. Why? Old Slow Mike does it for the challenge. "It's my only talent," he says. "I can put one foot in front of the other and keep going, slowly." He also loves the traveling to different states and enjoying the company of other runners. When he travels to a race he stays and visits the local attractions. He figures he has met over a thousand people he fondly calls his running buddies. And it's no wonder he has so many—Brooks is like a big cuddly bear in running shoes. He loves to chat with other runners and makes friends wherever he goes.

I asked him about his nutrition and training plan and to no surprise he doesn't follow either. "I don't have a nutrition plan unless you count the three beers a day I allow myself," he laughs. "I also don't follow any training plan. I used to train hard but now my knees are bone-on-bone so I do a lot of walking between races and even in races." He runs in pain, but he has a high level of tolerance. He wears two ID bracelets: a medical ID for his heart and another one that reads, "pain will go away but if you quit it will stay with you forever." "I just stay mentally focused," is his advice. Staying that focused doesn't come without a price. For instance, he promised to take his granddaughter to her high school dance but then the day of the dance his appendix ruptured. Not wanting to disappoint her, he went anyway and danced in excruciating pain before going to the emergency room for surgery. Then he ran a 5K the following weekend, definitely not recommended by his doctor. He did it anyway because he'd "already paid for it and at the end of the race they offer $1 Guinness. You'd have to be crazy to pass that up." His family medical chart has its share of cancers and heart issues so Brooks feels as if he is on borrowed time. "I thought I'd be dead by now but here I am so I might as well run more races." But to be prudent, he has all his papers in order for his wife, "just in case I drop dead at my next race."

His five-hundredth marathon in May of 2016 was a thrilling moment for Brooks. It was only six weeks after his surgery to replace a valve and his doctors were not happy with him, but come hell or high water, or drop dead on the course, Brooks was going to finish his five-hundredth marathon in Portland, Maine. He walked a "test" 5K three weeks after the surgery (which he did not tell his doctor about), and it didn't go well. When he finished the 5K he felt very dizzy and went to the EMT truck to have his blood pressure taken. It was 80 over 60 and they rushed him to the hospital. More tests showed that 50 percent of his kidneys had shut down. After that, he behaved himself so he could make it to the marathon.

The race director gave him clearance to start at 5:00 a.m. The race director also made him a special bib, #500. His wife followed him in her car along the course while his daughters prepared a celebration for him afterwards at the Great Lost Bear Tavern that features sixty beers on tap. "It was unbelievable," says Brooks. "My relatives all came, and five buddies of mine jumped in at mile 22 and ran with me to the finish." He was exhausted, finishing in eight hours and twenty-six minutes, but was so worth it? "To be honest, I didn't know if I would finish but I am so thrilled to have completed my five-hundredth marathon," says Brooks.

Since that marathon Brooks laments that his running has gone downhill. But for someone of Brook's stamina that doesn't mean much. Going downhill means that he ran three more marathons a week after his five-hundredth to finish his six-time 50 States Marathon Club venture. He had three southern states—South Carolina, Georgia, and Florida— which he finished in three days. He ran the Mainly Series of Marathons, as they don't have a cutoff time. In one, he came in last and won the Caboose Award. "I had to fight for last place," he laughs. "Fortunately the other runner dropped out." The last state will be Alaska, which he'll do in mid-2018 in Juno.

When I catch up with Brooks again in March of 2018, he asks me if he told me about his stroke. I would have remembered that so he proceeds to tell me how he suffered a stroke the previous November. It was right after he went in for a knee replacement in October of 2016. During the pre-surgery testing, the doctors found he had atrial fibrillation, irregular heartbeats that can lead to blood clots, stroke, heart failure, and other heart-related complications, and cancelled the surgery. A few days later, he ran a 5K race and felt terrible afterwards. He went home, sat down in his easy chair, and had a stroke. His wife came in the room, saw him listless in the chair, started pounding on his chest, and called 911. An ambulance arrived and he was admitted into the local hospital. An MRI scan showed a blood clot had entered his brain. He was immediately transferred to a Portland hospital thirty-five miles away where a neurosurgeon was waiting. According to Brooks, "He plucked that blood clot right out in no time and then zapped my heart back into rhythm."

After his post-surgery checkup, he asked the doctor if he could run Mount Washington in June 2018, a 7.5-mile run and the steepest course in all fifty states. The doctor cleared him. Other races for 2018 include a three-day race in May in New Jersey followed by the Oh Boy Marathon in Waterbury, Connecticut, and the Alaska Marathon in July. His total marathon count is up to 514.

He reflects on his running life and although it has been plagued with injuries, surgeries, a broken-down body, and a series of shots in his knee and back just so he can stand upright without pain, "I wouldn't trade it for the world," he says reflectively. "When I run I solve the problems of the world so I keep running because we have a lot of problems!" He's made so many friends through running and looks forward to seeing them even if it is once a year. Brooks is a favorite wherever he goes so it's no surprise that race directors always find a place for him. His running buddies are his extended family. His wife Denise, a former runner sidelined with injuries, comes to some events, but as he says, "There's nothing as boring as watching someone run." He knows he can depend on his buddies to show up, take care of each other, and have some beers afterwards.

The biggest motivator for Brooks is the fun of it. He also fundraises for Camp Sunshine, a retreat in Maine for children with life-threatening illnesses and their families. The program is free of charge to the families. Brooks has raised over $65,000 for the camp and tears up when he starts talking about it. Sometimes he has fun while fundraising. At his recent seven marathons in seven days in seven states event, which he did to raise money for Camp Sunshine, he wore a garter belt, the better for collecting dollars as he ran. One day he collected $166 in dollar bills. "The girls like to put it in the garter belt but the guys just hand it to me," he recalled. Many of the courses were loops which he enjoys as he gets to talk to more people. He's a terrific fundraiser and says that it's pretty easy when an old guy asks for money. He once asked someone to pledge ten bucks a mile. That didn't sound so bad until the person found out the race was three hundred miles.

Brooks has a big heart, is engaging, and deadpan funny. "My wife gets upset with me but knows better than to tell me not to run." He called her while she was away in Costa Rica and asked if she minded that he signed up for the Mount Washington race. She replied: "If you want to kill yourself go ahead." He tells me about his friend Julius who dropped dead at a race one hundred feet before the finish line. He was seventy-seven. After the funeral, Brooks and his running buddies, with the help of the local police, shut down the road leading up to those last one hundred feet of the course so that Brooks and all of Julius's running buddies could run across the finish line with his ashes so he would officially finish the race. The race director gave Julius's wife a finisher's medal. That's the kind of friend Brooks is.

At seventy-two, Brooks has twenty-two years of running under his belt. He feels his age and laughs that he really doesn't run marathons anymore, he walk/runs them with buddies. "When I was fifty, I Boston qualified [BQ] at my first marathon. Now, I couldn't BQ if my life depended on it. I'm twice as slow," he says. At first it was hard to accept when he slowed down in his sixties and then he had the heart surgery and then the stroke that almost brought him to his knees. "I have to accept the fact that I'm slow. I try as hard as I can and that's the best I can be. If I croak, I croak. I've had a great life. I won't be upset," he laughs. Just this year he's decided to cut his marathons to five a year plus one ultra, down from thirty-three a year. "I just can't do it anymore," he states. "I want to stay as healthy as I am now."

He receives lots of accolades and awards for his running and his fundraising but doesn't pay attention to them. He tells me one of his self-deprecating stories about getting a piece of mail from the Maine Senate. He thought it was junk mail and threw it out unopened. Then he read in his local newspaper how he received a certificate of merit from then Senator Olympia Snowe bestowing on him the Good Citizen of the Year Award. That was the "junk mail" he got rid of.

He's also a big supporter of veterans and served in the Maine National Guard for six years. When he ran the Bataan Death March, which honors the survivors of the 1942 Bataan March, a few remaining veterans of the march showed up. The runners got to shake hands with them at the start and then the vets at the finish saluted them. It was one of his most memorable races. When September 11 happened, he tried to enlist into the Marines, but at fifty, he was told he was too old.

Currently, he's working on his autobiography, *Beyond Badwater: One Thousand Races, One Thousand Places*. He sees it as a way of preserving his story for his grandchildren and friends.

Brooks has not only run more than a thousand races, he's lived a thousand lives. He tells me the time when he was fighting a fire and ran into a basement forgetting his breathing apparatus. He thought he wasn't going to make it out when another firefighter showed up and got him out. He still stays in touch with that firefighter to this day.

At the end of our final talk, I tell Brooks to behave himself and be careful out there. His reply sums up his attitude on life and running: "You gotta do what you gotta do. Suck it up, buttercup!"

Kevin Follett

DOB: March 10, 1961

Residence: Fort Collins, Colorado

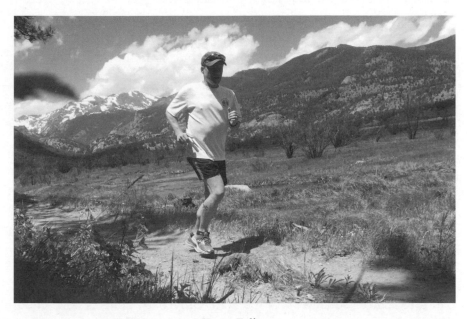

Kevin Follett

"100,000 miles and lions and tigers and bears."
Kevin Follett has recorded every mile he has run since January 1, 1973, when he was twelve years old. All those records, every day of them, are now available online on his blog. The vintage hand-written notes, charts, and photographs have been scanned into the digital age. There he is at thirteen, at his very first cross-country season standing with his

teammates, a skinny little guy at 4'10" and eighty pounds with blonde hair and a wide smile that seems to say "I love this!" You can see Follett running in high school with a determined look on his face, clocking a 5:45 mile as crosses the finish line. There he is at Kansas State University, where he lowers his mile time to 4:36. By September 1979, he has run 5,000. Moving forward to December 23, 2017, and you'll see a jubilant Follett at fifty-seven surrounded by family and friends celebrating his hundred-thousandth mile run. "Many people have asked me over the years, 'Why do you run?' Some of my answers might be: I was too small for football or basketball; it was something I was good at and enjoyed; I liked the feeling of endorphins after a run; I liked the challenge of seeing how far or fast I could go; etc. For whatever reason, it became an addiction, something that fit well with my compulsive behavior."

Follett was born in Fort Collins, Colorado. His dad was an agricultural professor at Colorado State University. Follett credits his father with encouraging him and then teaching him to start his running log. "My dad grew up poor. His family were ranchers and he lived up in the mountains. They didn't have any running water or electricity until 1953 when he went to college," says Follett. He can recall watching the 1972 Olympics on the family television with his dad and seeing Frank Shorter win gold in the marathon. "I wondered if I could ever run that far," he recalled. He didn't wait long to start finding out if running was his future. Outfitted in a new pair of Adidas running shoes, he joined his junior high cross-country team.

During the middle of junior high school in the spring of 1974, his dad took a professorship at Kansas State University. Follett's new school didn't offer cross country so he switched to track. The coaches weren't that knowledgeable about nutrition or great coaching advice as they had the team eat candy bars before meets, avoid water, and rest in the infield right before the meet. No warm-ups. "We all threw up after the race," he laughs. "I learned more about what not to do in training." Those middle school track seasons are what formed his desire to become a "good" high school coach later in life. After three seasons off from cross-country, he starts up again in high school. His training runs took him through cow pastures, over barbed wire and through the countryside of Kansas. He relished running outdoors in all weather.

On Christmas morning 1976, his dad gave him a calendar to log his miles. On January 1, 1977, he officially started his running log with paper and pencil, which continues to this day online. He logs his miles, his shoes, what animals he sees on his runs, and the weather. Pretty impressive for a fifteen-year-old. There's a photo from a meet in 1978 where the boys' cross-country team is wearing pink shorts even though the school colors were blue and white. When I ask him about that he laughs and says, "Oh yeah the pink? Our coach told us if we were tough enough to wear pink shorts we were tough enough to win."

While at Manhattan High School in Kansas, Follett and a group of his buddies formed their own running club, the Stickmen Running Club. They wrote a monthly newsletter and had shirts made up. In May of 1980 they decided to drive to Boulder, Colorado to run the second Bolder Boulder 10K and meet their idol, Frank Shorter. The night before the race they slept in the car and were rattled awake by the placement of the port-a-johns. They ran the race, which finished at the Boulder High School, and there standing in the middle of the field was Shorter. They boldly walked over, introduced themselves, and presented him with a Stickman Running shirt making him an honorable member. He didn't seem impressed. And yes, there is a photo of that event on the blog and Shorter does look aloof. The following year, Shorter came to Follett's town (Manhattan, Kansas) to run a 10K, which Follett also ran. After the race Follett went over to Shorter and asked for an autograph (apparently they forgot to get one when they gave him the T-shirt). Shorter looked up and said, "I remember you, you gave me that T-shirt. I love it, it's my favorite shirt."

After graduating high school—he was the valedictorian with a 4.0 average—he attended Kansas State, majoring in math, and ran cross country, making it to the nationals. He reached ten thousand miles his senior year and celebrated with a party at his fraternity. Instead of a keg, there was Gatorade. His accomplishment was written up in the local paper. The reporter asked him if he thought he would hit 100,000 and he responded it might take him forty years to reach that goal. He was off by three years.

By May of 1987, Follett was back in Fort Collins, a high school math teacher married to Karen, his college sweetheart and fast runner in her own right, and had just reached 25,000 miles. Follett was also managing a track team affiliated with a Christian organization, Campus Crusade for Christ, a team of high caliber university students that travel internationally to meets. International locations start entering the log.

Their baby daughter, Katie, was born at the end of year. It was a difficult birth and she almost didn't survive. Today, Katie is Katie Mackey, a Brooks-sponsored professional runner.

Follett keeps running and running. Nothing prevents him from reaching his goal. Not sub-zero temperatures, being hit by cars, chased by dogs, or being stranded on a glacier. In 1992 he ran his first 50K in brutal conditions and won the race setting a course record of four hours and sixteen minutes. In 1996 he reached 50,000 miles, logged in as "mile 50,000, August 15, Saratoga, Wyoming." He started coaching cross country at Fort Collins High School and took the team to his father's old ranch stead, now called Follett Ranch, to run and camp. By 2001, Katie was in seventh grade and started joining her dad on runs. Three other daughters have since joined the family and all became proficient runners.

Follett is as steady as a rock and gives thanks every day for his incredible life. But his years of running have come with a price—injuries. Over the years he's suffered a torn popliteal muscle in his left knee, chronically-tight IT bands, plantar fasciitis, and swelling in the sacroiliacs joint. In 1999 he tried to run through a stress fracture in his ankle, which only made it worse. For the first time since age twelve, he had to stop running and let it heal.

Family vacations are always outdoors and include running. There are hundreds of photos of Team Follett: Kevin, Karen, and their daughters, running in the woods, on beaches, in the mountains, basically, anywhere. Mile 75,000 was logged on March 25, 2007, in Rocky Mountain National Park. He carried a small camera with him on his runs to photograph the animals he saw on his runs. He came face-to-face with a black bear, ran into a mountain lion and her cubs—thankfully she backed away—and was attacked by a wild boar in a pineapple field in Hawaii that almost took off his leg. As harrowing as some of these encounters have been, Follett wouldn't trade one run. It's obvious that Follett not only loves being outdoors, he feels a connection to its beauty and its spiritual power.

In 2008 Follett coached his Fort Collins High School cross-country team to a state title. His daughter Kirsten was part of the winning team. Mile 80,000 was logged on April 11, 2009 at Horsetooth Reservoir in Colorado. He retired in 2011, which allowed him to spend more time traveling with his still-active Campus Crusade through

Christ team. Daughter Katie was running in Europe and they frequently crossed paths at meets. Follett became an unofficial regular at
the Brooks's events and training camps and was always greeted warmly
by the members. No doubt Katie had told them of her dad's quest to run
100,000. When icons of the sport such as Meb Keflezighi and Bernard
Legat came to the running camps to talk with the runners, they made
sure to have their picture taken with him and insisted on running a mile
with him so they would be on the list of "Follett's 100,000 Quest Running Partners." Two-time Olympian Nick Symmonds is also on the list
of Follett's Miles.

Mile 90,000 is run on July 30, 2013 in LaPorte, Colorado. Now
that he is closing in on his goal, he adds another: to run in all fifty states
before he reaches 100,000. He adds a column on his Excel sheet to track
the states. The other columns list his shoes and the animals he's seen.
Fifteen thousand deer to-date. He completed running in all fifty states
in May of 2015. The last four were all down South, which called for a
road trip. With Karen as his roadie, they drove from Georgia through
Alabama, on to Mississippi with a stop to visit Graceland, Elvis Presley's
home. The road trip ended in Tennessee as he checked off the last state.
Mile 95,000 was run on August 25, 2015, in Poudre Canyon, Colorado.

Follett can tell you in a split second what his monthly and yearly
mileage is: 203.3 a month and 2,400 per year. He is very precise. He
runs six days a week, taking Sunday off for church. He never did crazy
weekly mileage, keeping it at forty-five a week, maybe fifty. When the
kids were little he and Karen switched off watching them to get in their
runs. He drove the kids to school, "some of the best times I spent with
them," he recalls. When the girls were old enough to go on long runs
with him, he cherished their times together. "Some of the deepest and
most life-changing conversations take place on a run," says Follett.
"That's just one of the reasons I am so passionate about running. It has
enhanced my life beyond what I ever dreamed. I've gotten a lot out of
running over the years, and probably the best part was running with my
wife and daughters and having hours and hours to talk and grow closer."

Mile 99,000, which he reached on July 12, 2017, is very special
to Follett. To honor his dad, the man who inspired this quest by giving
him a small gift of a running log on Christmas Day when he was twelve
years old, he runs a mile through his father's hometown, Cowdrey, Colorado. The months and miles fly by, down to 999,997.

Approaching the milestone, Follett was filled with mixed emotions about his quest coming to closure—excitement, sadness, nervousness and uncertainty. He was nervous that he'd get sick in the last few days and not be able to complete it as scheduled. The plans for the event were already in motion. His entire family would be there, a rare occasion these days. So many friends asked to be involved, he was overwhelmed. "If I had just gone out and quietly run that hundred thousandth mile by myself, I would have been very sad," says Follett. "Being able to share this goal with so many others made it a completely different day, and it couldn't have turned out any better!"

On December 23, 2017, with three miles remaining, Follett and his family gathered with a group of friends at the Poudre Middle School in Laporte, Colorado, and ran along the Poudre River Trail. Thirty or more friends jumped in and out along the way. Custom bibs were made for everyone. News cameras were set up along the course. With a few yards to go, his daughters Katie and Kirsten ran ahead to hold up a finish line tape for their dad. Breaking the tape, Follett was all smiles. The forty-one-year quest was accomplished.

Follett is looking forward to the next phase of his running life when there won't be the pressure to log miles. He explains: "I knew that at some point, continuing to run as I had was unsustainable. For forty-one years I put in fifty miles a week. I am looking forward to continuing to run, but without the pressure to meet that goal." As a reward for his accomplishment, Follett purchased a road bike and mountain bike and enjoys exploring new places. But running will continue to be his main activity. He adds, "I don't know that anything else out there can replace the experience of a good run!"

He knows his accomplishment isn't extraordinary. There are many runners who have logged 100,000, even 200,000 or more miles. But what does make his particularly interesting is that he also logged his shoes, his running partners and every animal he saw while running for forty-one years. For example, 1,700 deer, 309 bald eagles, fourteen bears, five cougars, 130 alligators, and four dolphins. His log even includes elevation charts. He's run in all fifty states and twenty-two countries. And along the way he's inspired other runners with his dedication. As Follett says, "I'm just a regular guy who loves his family and loves to run."

Jeff Galloway

DOB: July 12, 1945

Residence: Atlanta, Georgia

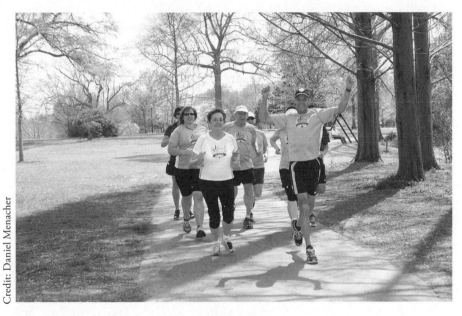

Credit: Daniel Menacher

Jeff Galloway

"Runners don't act their age."
Jeff Galloway transformed himself from an overweight thirteen-year-old to an Olympian through focused determination and dedicated training.

At Wesleyan University, Galloway was an All-American. Among his teammates were Amby Burfoot and Bill Rodgers. At the height of his career Galloway competed against some of the world's best athletes. At the 1972 Olympics he participated in the 10K and placed fourth at the Olympics marathon trials, behind Kenny Moore, Frank Shorter, and Jack Bacheler. He broke the US ten-mile record (47:49) in 1973 and has a six-mile best of 27:21. Among the races he has won are the Honolulu Marathon and the Atlanta Marathon. He was named by a recent USA Running poll as the most recognized person in the sport of running. For all his accomplishments, he is without ego. Now retired from professional running, he is best known for his signature Galloway Run Walk Method. He has coached more than a million runners and walkers to their goals through his program. What better coach to discuss how we can still reach our goals and even run PRs into old age?

Galloway spends just about every weekend traveling to race events where he is a sought-out speaker. I was fortunate to nail down a time when he was available to speak with me. What I gleaned from our conversation and in speaking to some of his former college track and cross-country teammates, as well as runners who swear by his method, is that Galloway is just about the humblest and kindest ambassador in the sport. His entire life has been dedicated to running in some way, whether he's writing about it in online newsletters, blogs, and more than twenty books, or talking about it in one of the approximately two hundred clinics that he conducts each year. He travels to a race event just about every weekend as a guest speaker.

John Franks "Jeff" Galloway was born in Raleigh, North Carolina. His father was in the navy and the family moved around quite a bit. Galloway had attended thirteen schools by the time he got to seventh grade. Due to the constant moving, he never had time to get involved in sports programs and became sedentary, gaining weight. "I was the last one picked when choosing up sides for games," he says. His father retired from the navy when he was thirteen, and he was finally able to stay in a school long enough to participate on a sports team. He chose track not because he was good at it, but because the kids were funny and accepted him. That social aspect was just as important to him as the running. The weight came off and he realized he was good at running. In high school he became the state champion in the two-mile.

After college he spent three years in the navy, stationed on a ship in Vietnam. When he left the navy he attended graduate school at Florida State University, where he met his future wife Barbara, who is a fast runner in her own right. In Florida, Galloway started training with Frank Shorter and Jack Bacheler in preparation for the 1972 Olympics. Bacheler had started the Florida Track Club, and Galloway and Shorter were members. All three made the Olympic team that year, Shorter and Bacheler in the marathon and Galloway in the 10,000 meters. He could have made the marathon team, but he helped his friend Bacheler, who had run the 5,000 meters for the US team at the 1968 Mexico City Olympics, secure a spot instead. Here's how that happened: Galloway and Shorter had already qualified for the Olympic team at 10,000 meters the week before. Bacheler also ran the 10,000 meters at the Trials but didn't make the team. Galloway was at peak training for the marathon, his preferred event, but he wanted his friend to be part of the 1972 Olympics and prepared to give up his spot for Bacheler. His plan was to pace Bacheler, stay steady, and aim for third place behind Shorter and Kenny Moore, who were out in front for most of the race. But at mile 21, Bacheler started slowing down and struggled. Galloway stuck with his friend, and through encouragement, sheer will, and expert cheerleading, kept him on pace. They entered the stadium neck and neck and the crowd went wild. At the last second, Galloway stepped back and let Bacheler finish in front of him, ceding third place on the 1972 Olympic team. "Helping my friend make the team was and still is one of the greatest joys of my career," Galloway says. That's just one example of why runners flock to Galloway at events, standing in line for hours. His calming manner and soft southern tone reassures even those with the worst cases of the jitters that they can succeed.

After the Olympics, Galloway and Barbara settled in Atlanta, Georgia and founded Phidippides, one of the first specialty running stores in the country, but over time it wasn't profitable. To keep the doors open, Galloway, a savvy businessman, started offering coaching services, running camps, and retreats. His elite running friends came along as guest speakers. "People loved it," he says. "For the first time, they were engaging their brains, not just their feet, in learning how to run." He offered a class in beginning running and realized that to keep these newbies injury-free as they learned to run—and to enjoy running—he needed to insert walking breaks in the training. At the end of the ten-week session, the group ran their first 5K or 10K and no one had injuries. That became his blueprint for the Galloway Run Walk Method. And the store is still open.

One of the key issues for being successful with Galloway's method is acknowledging ego, especially for longtime runners who were nurtured on the belief that walking has no place in a running program. Galloway gets kudos from more than 300,000 runners of all ages who believe his method works and saves wear and tear on the body. There is scientific research behind his program. "This isn't something I just came up with on a whim," he says. "It's based on a cognitive strategy to retrain the subconscious brain to avoid anxiety and burnout." He and Barbara put in months of training on their own, tweaking the run/walk ratios. And they are the proof. After years of hard-pounding professional running, Galloway, at seventy-three, runs a marathon a month and has been doing that for some time. That's twelve marathons each year, for a total of more than 220 to date. And he's never injured. In fact, he feels great. He goes out for a recovery run the day after a marathon, which he was never able to do when he was running in his prime years. And in his humble way, he says he's not amazing, just an average Joe who found the right way to run forever. "I think the people I see at races are the ones who are amazing," he says. "It's the seventy-, eighty-, and even ninety-year-olds who are running marathons and feeling great at their age."

Besides the Run Walk Method, Galloway also adheres to the basic marathon training principles: putting in the months of training, being dedicated to your goal, and finding a mantra that works. He's a big believer in mental training. "Find that magic word that keeps you going," he says. "Words like 'I can' should be at the forefront of the brain." When his clients have injuries or a layoff from running, he advises the following: "When mature runners start back after an extended layoff I recommend only walking for the first two weeks, gradually increasing the distance of the walk, using a gentle stride. I recommend easing back into running with a slow jog or "shuffle" for five to fifteen seconds, followed by a thirty- to sixty-second walk. Gradually increase and back off if there are aches and pains. During the layoff period you've most likely lost a good deal of your physical ability to run, but not the memory. Be patient. Stay below your normal threshold in the beginning weeks. The biggest risk in coming back is compensating for the injury site—the weak link—with an abnormal gait, and then you risk getting injured again."

There are two points he is especially emphatic about: speed kills, and stretching has no benefit. "As we age, speed is the number-one cause of injury," he says. And he doesn't recommend stretching, has never done it and has never read any study that proves it is beneficial. And he isn't a big proponent of running for time. "If you run for the clock, eventually you will get injured," he says. "Run for the sheer enjoyment of it and it will reward you tenfold."

Galloway digs deep and does a lot of research on the topic of running and its benefits. During our talk, he refers to a book he is thoroughly enjoying and learning from, *The Story of the Human Body: Evolution, Health, and Disease* by Daniel Lieberman, a Harvard professor of human evolution. In the book, there is a chapter entitled "Disuse: Why We are Losing It by Not Using It," where Lieberman states: "Human bodies were not designed like the Brooklyn Bridge but instead evolved to grow by interacting with their environment . . . every body needs appropriate, sufficient stresses to tune its capacities." The old adage, "no strain, no gain" is profoundly true. How many times have we heard that phrase as we age? Galloway also refers to a study from a 2016 University of Arizona research team that revealed runners' brains have greater functional connectivity than the brains of more sedentary individuals. The study compared brain scans of young adult cross-country runners to a group of young adults who didn't engage in regular physical activity. The scan focused within several areas of the brain, including the frontal cortex, which is important for cognitive functions such as planning, decision-making, and the ability to switch attention between tasks. The results showed that the runners' brains had greater functional connectivity than those of the more sedentary group, and that this led to better attitudes, higher energy levels, and increased critical thinking.

According to Galloway, "The key to running until you're one hundred is to maintain good health and nutrition, stay within your capabilities, and exercise regularly enough to maintain the adaptations you've worked hard to achieve. Age-appropriate training allows you to enjoy running more while reducing aches and pains.

"I don't feel any different today than I did in my twenties," says Galloway. "Age is just a number, and runners never act their age. When I meet runners at events and clinics regardless of their age, I see a group of runners with vitality, mental sharpness, and a love for life. That's the gift of running."

Talking with Galloway is refreshing and uplifting. He truly makes you feel you can do anything, run anywhere for any distance, and run for life if you follow his advice, which is to be patient with injuries, take baby steps in getting back to running, and not to listen to the ego. His times have fallen off, but he doesn't give that a thought. He's had his share of wins and medals. Now it's all about running for the sheer joy of it and for life. He recently ran a marathon with a ninety-year-old and found him as sharp as the thirty-year-olds he meets at events. He sums up his philosophy on the aging process: "Age is a number. The body won't let you down if you take care of it. How you age is a choice, so make the right ones." That's sound advice.

Julian Gordon

DOB: February 10, 1936

Residence: Lake Bluff, Illinois

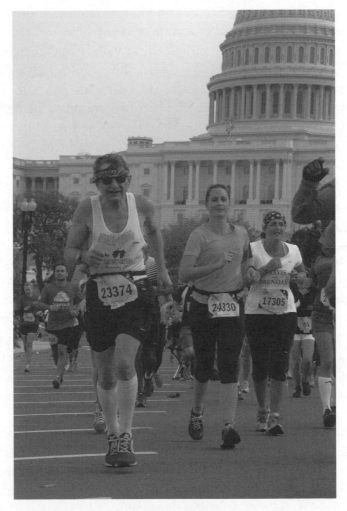

Julian Gordon

"I'm just happy to still be running."
At the age of eighty-two, Julian Gordon is still running marathons. Gordon, a PhD biophysicist and adjunct professor of biomedical engineering at Northwestern, became serious about running at the age of fifty-two and averages three marathons a year. He led the 2017 Chicago Marathon 5:10-pace group and brought them all home on time. His philosophy on aging and losing speed is simple: "I get slower every year but I was never fast to start with so it makes it easier to accept."

Gordon was born in London before World War II. By 1939, his father had realized that London was no longer safe and moved the family to the countryside. Gordon was three at the time and can recall sitting on packing boxes eating puffed wheat wondering where they were going. They moved to High Wycombe, thirty miles outside London. His father's decision was preemptive, as shortly after they moved a decision was made to evacuate all children in London. If he had waited, Gordon and his brother would have been removed from their parents. It's one of many moments that Gordon refers to as a serendipitous decision that would form his life.

After the war his family returned to London where he finished high school. When he was applying to primary school at age seventeen, his teachers were toting Oxford and Cambridge as the only schools to attend for a bachelor's degree. Gordon was turned down at both schools, although he was an A-level student and the first from his high school to receive a state scholarship for a fully-funded college education. "It appeared that I had no future," said Gordon in his still-noticeable soft English accent. He decided to attend King's College London as his brother was already enrolled there studying law. He selected a major in special physics as he had always been interested in the subject, but he admits that he had no concept of science as a career, what kind of work a scientist actually did, and had never known a scientist. Yet another example of his serendipitous journey through life.

Over the course of his career as a scientist, Gordon has made groundbreaking contributions. His work led to the first home pregnancy test. He was responsible for inventing the Western Blot, an important method used today in molecular biology, biochemistry, and immunogenetics for the characterization and detection of proteins. These were busy years for Gordon, working twenty-four hours in a lab, no time for exercise, and smoking heavily. "I was in terrible shape," recalls Gordon, then thirty-six.

"I knew this was bad for my health, but I couldn't quit the smoking." He finally quit when his first child was born. He moved from New York to Switzerland shortly thereafter and took advantage of the beautiful trails and hills to start jogging with his dog on gorgeous mountain trails on Sunday mornings. It became his routine. He'd map out a new trail every week and then meet his family at a quaint mountain village café for breakfast. He felt himself getting stronger and loved the feeling. He kept this up for several years until he moved to Illinois in 1984.

In Lake Bluff, he met other runners and was surprised that people actually ran more than once a week. He joined the Lake Forest-Lake Bluff running club and fell into it with zeal. He entered his first race, a 5K. "I didn't do well, finished in the lower half," he remembers. But he loved the camaraderie and being part of the running scene. Although not fast, he had endurance. He upped the distance, running 10Ks, half marathons, and finally in 1996 ran his first marathon, at age fifty-one. The idea to run the Chicago Marathon came from his son who was a good runner, in great shape, and thought it would be fun to run with his dad. But by the time the marathon came around, his son was injured so Gordon ran it by himself. "It was hell!" he claims. "I swore I would never do that again." Three months later he was planning his next one. Then another one and another one, and now he's at seventy-six marathons and counting. He tried a triathlon once but says, "That was a bad idea." He doesn't do ultras, claiming his body can only handle 26.2 miles.

Gordon approaches his running like a scientist. He doesn't do it for the passion or the exhilaration, although he feels that. He does it out of curiosity. "I approach everything in my life with the question, *I wonder what would happen if,*" he says. His best time is 3:45, but that's in a steep decline. "I'm just happy I'm still out there," says Gordon. "If I can stay above the fiftieth percentile, I'm having a good run." But he's noticed a new phenomenon; as he gets older and slower, he is actually winning his age group. "I've become competitive at this age and I like it," he laughs. "If I don't take first age I get upset."

When he turned seventy-five in 2011, Gordon won first in his age group at the Journeys Marathon in Eagle River, Wisconsin, as well as at the Anchorage Mayor's Marathon and the Marine Corps Marathon. When Gordon ran MCM in 2012, he won his age division by an hour. Sometimes he has stiff competition and at other times he is the only one in his age group. "It's so rewarding to win, or even place in races," he adds. "Simply exhilarating for me." He took second age at the London Marathon in 2015. His older brother also inherited the running gene as he has a thirty-five-year streak at the London Marathon.

His running took on new meaning when he became a pacer at the 2001 Chicago Marathon. His first year, he led the 3:50 group, which he personally needed to qualify for Boston. He missed the mark by four minutes. Looking back he realizes that was a stupid move, putting his own goals first. The following year and every year since he has brought his group in on the mark. Chicago prides itself on its pace leaders' ability to bring their group in on time. Paul Miller runs the pace leader teams at Chicago and has been working with Gordon for eleven years. Miller has nothing but praise for his favorite octogenarian pacer: "Julian's been a part of the team for as long as I can remember. He is a kind soul who is very generous with his time and encouragement for his fellow runners. Two of the endearing qualities I've witnessed in Julian are patience and persistence. Turns out both are required to be a reliable pacesetter!"

Ever the scientist, Gordon has his own system for pacing his groups. "I carry a sign with the pace time on it," Gordon said. "On the back, I write the time we need to achieve after each mile. If we're a little behind, I pick it up the next mile. If we're ahead, I slow down a little." He also creates his own spreadsheet with the mile pace on it, which he attaches to the stick he is carrying and refers to as needed. He encourages his group to talk and inspire one another to achieve their common goal. Gordon also speaks five languages so he can converse with many runners in their own language. When the going gets tough, he reassures his group how great they will feel when they cross the finish line and fulfill their dream. He's thought of relinquishing his pace leader spot as he feels he is getting too old for it, but he keeps getting invited back.

On a perfect day he can still run a five-hour marathon. In 2016 he ran Grandma's in 5:10, taking first in his age. "It was a hot day, and I think I could have done better but the weather did me in," he explains. "I wither in the heat." His most recent biggest claim to fame was at the 2013 Marine Corps Marathon where at age seventy-seven he ran a 4:55, taking first in his age and beating the second place by more than an hour.

Asked how running has played a part in his life and how it has fused with the science part of his brain, he responds: "Running is huge for my self-esteem. I am much more confident in every other aspect of my life because of my running. My wife thinks I am on an ego trip with my running accolades, but so what!" he laughs. "Being at peak health condition I can focus on original ideas, solve intricate problems, and concentrate longer. I can stay awake longer and am more alert due to my . running and conditioning."

Running has also brought him closer to his family. When his kids were young, he spent long hours in the lab. Now, he enjoys running and taking backpacking trips with his son. Several years ago they spent weeks together in Yosemite backpacking the trails. His son recently received his physician's assistant degree and during his studies, read articles written by his father. Gordon was delighted when his son called him to say, "Dad, I finally understand what you did all those years in the lab!" Gordon is equally proud of his daughter, an accomplished percussionist in New York.

He runs five miles a day, five times a week. When training for a marathon he'll add long runs of twenty miles on the weekends. "I don't necessarily follow a program." He adds, "I just run how I feel." He's thought of quitting marathons but ultimately finds it too rewarding. "I don't want to be the dinosaur that doesn't know enough when it is time to quit," he explains. "But on the other hand, I want to take full advantage of my running as long as I can. It's part of my serendipitous philosophy of life. I'll keep running 'til I come up with a reason not to." His 2018 marathon schedule suggests he's not ready to quit just yet. In May, he ran the Eagle River Marathon in Wisconsin, which he has done every year since its inception. In June 2018, he ran the Charlevoix Marathon in Michigan, and then he was a pace leader for Chicago in October, and will compete New York City Marathon in November.

Not only is Gordon not retiring from running any time soon, he started a new job. In 2005, he retired from Abbott Laboratories after twenty-five years and is now the chief scientific officer of Inspirotec, a startup company. He is working on a device that determines which allergens are in the air in a persons' home or another location so they can take the necessary steps for relief. "We turned it into a marketable product," Gordon said. "We put the device in their home. They send it into the lab and we analyze it for allergens.

"Running contributes to living a meaningful life as I grow older," Gordon says. "You have to keep mentally and physically fit to enjoy the aging process." When I ask him his thoughts on the new-age marketing term "anti-aging" plastered on just about everything from face creams to antioxidants, he responds: "I don't worry about terms like anti-aging. Anyone can define a term and use it for whatever rubbish they might think fit. But anti-aging that promises to reverse aging is at the best puffery, at the worst fraud. I don't think aging can be reversed. The best thing to do is to maintain vigorous physical and mental health to minimize the effects of aging." Spoken like the scientist he is.

His personal motto also sums up his philosophy on life: *Mens sana in corpore sana*, which translated means "A sound mind in a sound body." We finish the interview with a question. I ask him to describe his perfect day: "My perfect day is a five-mile run to the beach and back in crisp but sunny weather. After that I can deal with whatever life will throw at me and end up laughing."

Harold Green

DOB: April 14, 1945

Residence: Suffern, New York

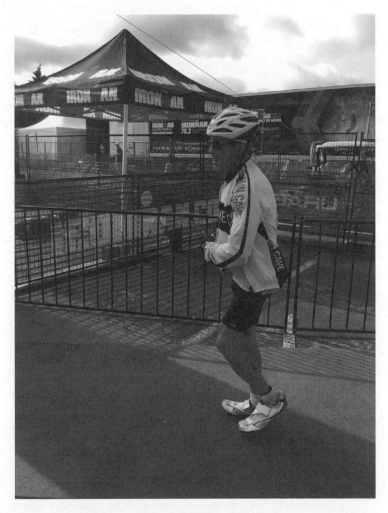

Harold Green at the 2017 Mount Tremblant Ironman.

A Life Fulfilled.

When Harold Green decides to do something, he goes big. He started running at sixty-two to cope with his wife's terminal cancer and ran his first marathon at sixty-five. Six months later he did another marathon and qualified for the Boston Marathon. At age seventy, he did his first Ironman. To date, at age seventy-three, he has completed three full Ironmans, a number of half Ironmans and six marathons. There is no stopping Green. "I always feel great when I cross the finish line because it means I'm not dead yet," says Green.

Green grew up in Beacon, New York, a small upstate town of five-square miles, sixty miles north of Manhattan. His parents, conservative Jews, did not allow him to play sports on Saturday, which ruled out most team sports. So instead, he joined the band. "Running in those days wasn't a major event like it is today. I didn't know anyone who ran distance races and the first Ironman event wasn't even organized until 1978," recalls Green. "But I rode my bike everywhere through town. That's how we got around, on our bikes."

At Temple University, Green took up intramural sports but "didn't even break a sweat." It was more for social fun. He was a serious student and grades came first. He went on to get his masters' degree in education and taught chemistry in Wappingers Falls, New York. By 1969 he was married to his college sweetheart, also a teacher, and they moved to nearby Monsey. Two kids later, his life was pretty much structured. At thirty-five, he joined a gym to get in shape but admits it was also a social outlet. "I did more talking and schmoozing with other members than I did reps," laughs Green.

In 2008 his wife was diagnosed with adrenal cancer. He realized he needed to get in better shape so he could take care of her as well as himself throughout the long terminal illness. He took up running because "it was an easy outlet." A running buddy challenged him to run a marathon, and not one to turn down a challenge, he jumped on it. At sixty-five, he ran his first marathon, the 2010 New Jersey Marathon. He was still working at the time so rose early to get in his weekday runs and did long runs on the weekends. He finished the marathon in 5:38. The day was blistering hot, with temperatures in the nineties. He was thrilled just to finish. On the way home he got mad at himself for his time. "I wanted to do better," he recalls. The competitive juices started to flow.

He joined a running club, trained hard, and six months later ran the New York City Marathon in 4:13 and qualified for the Boston Marathon. But there was a catch. He missed the sign-up window. Desperate to run Boston—"I qualified, damn it!"—he looked into other avenues and found out he could run for a charity for $5,000. He couldn't justify spending that sum with his wife's medical bills. One day at his gym, he was complaining about the $5,000 when a man in the locker room overheard the conversation and out of the blue offered to pay the $5,000.

Six months later he ran the 2011 Boston Marathon, his third marathon in his first year of taking up running. Conditions were brutal that year with the temperatures reaching 88 degrees. Runners were offered a deferment for the following year but Green decided to run. "I didn't know when I would ever get in again," he laughs. He finished in 5:30 despite the heat.

He was just getting the knack of marathoning when he decided to take up triathlons. At sixty-seven, he was the oldest finisher at his first sprint distance event. When Green's wife was first diagnosed, he bought her a book about visiting all the fifty states thinking it would be a fun, distracting goal. By 2012 they had eight states left and they decided to make it their quest to see them. Her doctor thought it was a great idea, although by that time she was so frail and ill that she could barely get in and out of a car. They completed their goal but then decided to go back to their favorite places. In August of 2013, they drove to Lake Placid for the weekend. The Lake Placid Ironman (IMLP) had just taken place in July, and the signs were still up all over town. Green was mesmerized by the endurance race and decided to do IMLP the following year. That night, he booked the hotel room and signed up with a charity team to get entry. His wife was happy for him, telling him to "go for it!" She passed away the following month.

He had eleven months to train for the grueling endurance race, but while out on a training ride he crashed on his bike and tore his shoulder tendons. He was able to defer his entry to the following year and completed his first Ironman in 2015 with a time of 16:30 at age seventy. He describes it as the most difficult thing he has ever done. He struggled on the hilly bike course and fumbled through the transitions. Being a positive person, he also wanted to enjoy the event and not "fall on my sword in defeat." He recalls running the marathon in slow motion. But finish he did and he was jubilant. By the time he crossed the finish line he was drained, dehydrated, and exhausted. He wandered over to the medical tent requesting an IV of fluids. The medics took his vitals, told him he was fine, gave him a coke, and threw him out of the tent.

He got hooked on the Ironman and vowed to train harder for the next one. A year later he came back to Lake Placid and finished in 15:45, bettering his time. Three months later he completed Ironman Louisville and finished in 15:06. His friends and kids think he is crazy and run through all the scenarios that could happen to him. "Yes, it could all happen," he acknowledges. "But I know what to expect, I train well, and I love it. Life is short so do what you love. I am grateful to be at any start line."

At seventy-two, he didn't slow down. As Green describes his year, I am exhausted just listening to him. We are sitting in a neighborhood café. Green has just come from a hot yoga workout and is wearing a black T-shirt that reads, "Pain Cave." He is engaging, fun to talk with, and a charmer. I ask him if he is dating and he says with a twinkle that he has lots of girlfriends. It's easy to see why. He's a catch, but with a caveat. All his friends are runners or tri-athletes and any companion has to embrace that life. He kicked off 2017 with the Disney Dopey Challenge, a 5K, 10K, half, and full marathon in a single weekend. Due to bad weather the organizers canceled the half but Green completed the 5K in 35:00, the 10K in 1:09, and the marathon in 5:57. Six months later in June he entered a half Ironman in Syracuse, New York. The temperature hit 93 degrees and things turned ugly. He wanted to quit but kept going because his daughter attended Syracuse University and he wanted to get the medal for her. It took a toll on him. He was depleted mentally and physically at the end. But he still entered the August Mount Tremblant Ironman and for the first time he had to quit. "I couldn't do it—I bonked," he laments.

Although he made the right decision to quit, he was angry with himself. He needed redemption and signed up for a half Ironman in North Carolina in August. Among all his qualities, Green is also relentless. He has the stamina and energy of a forty-year-old. At the half Ironman, he takes third in his age. While standing on the podium, the announcer says that the first and second finisher gets a spot to the 2018 Half Ironman World Championship in South Africa. The second place finisher leans over to Green and says he can't go and would he like his spot. "I'll take it!" he tells me. He finished 2017 with the Philadelphia

Marathon. It was a miserable day with winds gusting at 40 miles per hour. He didn't put in a lot of training and despite heavy rain and winds he finished in 4:57.

For the World Championships in September of 2018, the first time an Ironman World Championship event will be held on the African continent, Green hired a coaching team. He also has a cadre of friends who will also be on hand to support and encourage him. Ever since he took up triathlons and running he has given back to all his friends who have supported him. Doing your first triathlon? Green will be there. Doing your first Ironman? Green will be your Sherpa. During the 2016 Ironman in Maryland, the weather was so bad that the swim was cancelled and the bike was cut short. High winds and flooding were a major factor. Green went to the event to help out friends. He waded through knee-high water to support them on the run. He braved the winds and flooding to be with them as much as possible. That's what Green does for his friends, who for the most part are half his age. "We help each other," says Green.

When I ask him about his 2017 Thanksgiving plans, he tells me he spent the day feeding the homeless and then had dinner with his kids and grandkids. "Time and health is our most precious commodity and I plan to fill my days with both," he adds. He knows he has been lucky to avoid injuries with the exception of the torn shoulder from the bike crash. He stretches every day, loves his hot yoga, and meditates every morning. He prefers triathlons to the marathon as they are easier on the body. He explains: "In a marathon I am pounding pavement for five or more hours. In a triathlon, even an Ironman, the swim is non-impact, and I can coast on the bike on the downhills. By the time I get off the bike, I can't wait to run."

He tries to convince me that what he does isn't crazy. I'm not sure about that. He tries to convince me that because he came to endurance sports late in life his body is fresh. Maybe I think he's crazy because he puts me to shame. I can't imagine keeping his grueling race schedule. He is taking a course in functional medicine with the goal to get certified to teach it. (Functional medicine determines how and why illness occurs by addressing the root of the cause of the disease and restores health through nutrition and lifestyle.) He'll be great at this.

When he has two seconds to spare, Green explains to me why he is so active. "I appreciate every minute of every day. As I get older I want to make sure that I am self-reliant, that I don't end up in a nursing home with a pile of bills and become a burden to my kids. I am mindful of my lifestyle, what I eat, how I exercise, and also make time to socialize. Those three things are key to my life and keep me happy, healthy, and content." He's learned to meditate, which wasn't easy, but he does it every morning. He's adopted two rescue cats, which he gets a kick out of. Walking through Ridgewood with Green is like being with a celebrity. Everyone knows him. This is the town where he hangs out and is like an unofficial mayor. He greets everyone with a bear hug and a smile.

A perfect day for Green starts with a shot of espresso, followed by a swim, followed by a healthy breakfast of granola with yogurt or eggs. Then a two-hour bike ride followed by a nap. After the nap, a leisurely three-mile run. Then he catches up with friends and family, grills some fish for dinner with a glass of wine and calls it a day. Harold Green is a happy man. His life is fulfilled. The one tip he tells everyone is to enjoy the day. "Life is a precious commodity. Time and health is all we have."

William Gross

DOB: September 29, 1953

Residence: Ridgefield, Connecticut

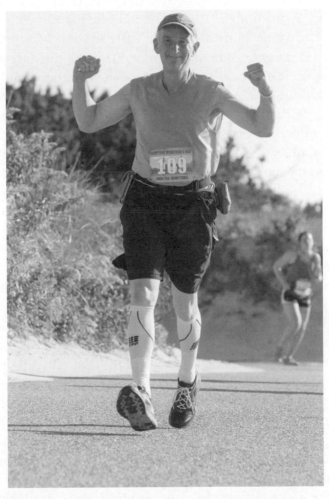

Bill Gross on the way to completing his one-hundredth marathon.

"Redefining aging."

Bill Gross took up running at age fifty. Now sixty-four, he has run 103 marathons in a span of fourteen years, an average of eight a year with no injuries. He officially became Marathon Maniac #686 in 2007. (To become an official Marathon Maniac you must, at the very lowest entry level, run two marathons within sixteen days or three marathons within ninety days. To be in the top echelon of Maniacs you must run a marathon every weekend of the year.) Gross has embraced his running life with a passion that is infectious. Sitting in his office in Connecticut, he shows me his favorite marathon memorabilia. There's a gold USATF Phidippides Award from 2010, one of eight he has earned, for his numerous participation in road races; his 2013 Boston Marathon medal, which still brings a choke in his throat; a 2018 wall calendar with April 16 already blocked out for this year's Boston Marathon; and the 2007 Goofy Award for running Disney World Half Marathon and Marathon back to back. "Running has enriched my life beyond what I ever imagined," says Gross. "Every time I go to the starting line of a race, I know how lucky I am."

Gross grew up in a suburb of Philadelphia in what he describes as a traditional middle-class family. His father worked retail at Gimbels Department Store, and his mother was a stay-at-home mom. In high school he preferred solo sports like golf, skiing, and singles tennis. Recalls Gross, "I was tall but uncoordinated so I wasn't good at team sports like basketball." He credits his mother with instilling in him a love for tennis. She played competitively up until age seventy-five and inspired in him a competitive nature for winning. "I feel her presence when I run my marathons," says Gross.

After graduating from Boston University in 1976, he went into advertising, working for the big firms such as J. Walter Thompson, Benton & Bowles, and Grey Advertising and worked on campaigns for some of the industry's largest advertisers such as Unilever, Kraft, Nestlé, Pepsi, and Procter & Gamble. At Benton & Bowles, while working in the media department, he shared a cubicle with a very attractive and opinionated young lady who "I fought with on a daily basis," and is now his wife of thirty-four years. They lived in Brooklyn, where Gross recalls he would wake up on a particular Sunday morning in November and see thousands of people running and wonder why they were all out so early in the morning. Life was good for Gross. He and his wife had a daughter, he was happy and successful at work, and he played lots of golf.

At the height of his career, he took a position in Los Angeles and commuted every week, boarding a flight Monday morning out of New York and returning home Friday night. "It became a routine, but not a healthy one for me or my family," recalls Gross. He was there on the morning of September 11, 2001. "I watched the Towers fall while in my hotel room," he said of that day. It took him five days to get a flight home and he can still recall the smell of burning ash and embers that hung in the air over Manhattan and filtered into the plane. It was a life-changing moment for him, as it was for so many people. He quit his job to spend more time with his wife and daughter and to plan a more meaningful life for himself, something that would give back to society in a positive way. His other reason for a life-changing event was his health. He had ballooned to 235 pounds. "Weight gain is an interesting thing," says Gross. "It creeps up on you and then one day you look in the mirror and ask what happened?" He wanted to get his health back not only for himself but for his family. "I wanted to be here for my daughter and at the rate I was going, I was not on a good track."

With a longtime friend, he opened the Brookfield Learning Center in 2002, a place for students, elementary through high school, who need help with their homework, preparing for tests, etc. "This was my redemption for all sugary cereals and Kool-Aid we pushed on kids," he laughs. He also joined a gym and worked with a personal trainer. The weight dropped and the fitness kicked in. Within a year, he weighed 149 pounds and friends thought he was sick, but he felt great. He started running on a treadmill and worked up to his first 5K. He went from thinking he would finish last ("What time does the course close?" he recalls asking) to feeling a latent competitive streak as he passed people on the course. He placed second in his age group (he was fifty) and became obsessed with running and getting faster. "I became obsessed with my time," says Gross. "Running lends itself to the Type A personality who wants to shave seconds or minutes off a previous time."

His next race was the Ridgefield Half Marathon and then he was ready for the big time. In 2003, he ran the Philadelphia Marathon, his first, in 3:59:58 (two seconds under his goal time). That was the defining moment of his marathon career. "I was hooked," he describes. "I started shopping marathons and signing up like a maniac." In 2004, he ran the Chicago Marathon (3:54) and three weeks later ran the Marine Corps Marathon (4:11). In 2005, he ran three marathons in three months. Then he ran eight to ten a year, until he reached one hundred. His only injury came early in 2004, and it wasn't even running related. (He hit his leg on a coffee table.)

For the next thirteen years Gross ran marathons all over the world. Combining running with travel is a big motivator for him. "My wife and I have always enjoyed and made time for travel but running gave me a new perspective on cities such as Rome, Venice, and Paris where I ran marathons or just heading out for a morning run in Ireland, London, or Tuscany," says Gross. He was in Berlin on business in 1989 the week the Wall came down and returned twenty-one years later to run the marathon where there was no trace of a wall. He ran through New Orleans on a new seawall after Katrina in 2005 and on the New Jersey shore where Sandy swept away the boardwalks in 2012 and re-routed the course. "These are all things I experienced as a runner," he says. One of his most memorable marathon travels combined the Venice Marathon and his sixtieth birthday, returning to the city where he married his wife.

He wanted his hundredth marathon to be Philadelphia where it all started in 2003 but he got nervous that something would derail his efforts. So without telling anyone he signed up for the Hamptons Marathon a month before Philadelphia and ran it without a hitch. After the marathon he drove over to Sag Harbor on Long Island where he used to spend childhood summers with his mother. Regrettably, she was taken by cancer before Bill ran his first marathon. He walked the beach and thanked her for giving him the competitive spirit all those years ago to go for the goal. Then he was ready to run Philadelphia, which turned out to be number 101.

Gross has enjoyed the luxury of being injury-free. "My knees are young," he laughs. He's worked with a trainer for more than ten years fine-tuning his cross training and his diet. He can bench press more than two hundred pounds and do a 120-pound bicep curl. Not shabby for a sixty-four-year old.

To explain how he stays motivated after running 103 marathons, he breaks them down into three segments. The first twenty-five were driven by an obsessive streak to run under four hours or to place in his age group. If he was two minutes off his goal time, he considered it a failure. "I was driven by data and numbers," he explains. "It was so new to me and I wanted to be a success." The second twenty-five were harder. As he slowed down in his late fifties, he had a difficult time adjusting so he shifted the goal. Now he was running to maintain his health, accepting the fact that he was older but still able to enjoy marathons. "It was difficult at first but I finally found a way to enjoy the day and not feel disappointed afterward," explains Gross. "I developed an appreciation for the event and was happy to be there."

In his sixties, he shifted the goal again. Now, he enjoys being out on the course, finally looking at the scenery along the way and socializing with other runners. He always finishes even if it takes five hours. "I'd rather explain a slower time than not finishing at all," he explains. He picked that tidbit up from Bill Rodgers, one of his running heroes. He attended an expo where Rodgers was speaking and asked him how he deals with not winning anymore. Rodgers explained that it was really hard not to be competitive and at the top any longer. In order not to lose his motivation for staying in the game, he had to change his expectations. Now, he runs because he still has that passion but the goal has shifted from winning outright to winning his age division.

At sixty-four, Gross is adopting Rodgers's goal. He is switching to running half-marathons where he feels he can compete in his age division. "I still have that competitive edge," he says with a laugh. "I can start making my charts again and filling in the data to see what time I need to beat to win." Then he turns philosophical: "Running has given me a second life. People ask me when I am going to retire. My response is always, why? From what? I am still productive. Our parents at our age were already in Florida sitting on their rockers and waiting for mahjong to start. That's not who I am or how I see our generation as a whole." He points out that most of the literature on aging in our society seems patronizing and the general advice is to accept the decline. The best we can hope for is to delay the unavoidable. As a runner, Gross finds this view unacceptable. "I have never met a committed runner with that perspective. Our generation is looking for achievable challenges, activities that we may not have had the time or money to pursue up until now. Staying healthy is a great byproduct but infrequently the ultimate goal. Look at the older runners at the finish line of a marathon. Is their sense of achievement any less profound than younger runners? I would argue the opposite. They see their success in a broader context based of life experience."

Gross is one of many senior runners who are changing the face of aging in our society. He is living the words of Dylan Thomas: "Do not go gentle into that good night. Old age should burn and rave at close of day/Rage, rage against the dying of the light." He is too content and happy to rage but he is making a difference in his own quiet way. While we are at his office, a week before Christmas, former high school students who studied there for SATs and other prep courses and are now in college stop in to say hello. They greet Gross with smiles and handshakes and ask about his marathons. They are obviously in awe of their gray-haired tutor. And why shouldn't they be? He is setting an example to follow your dreams regardless of age or ability. And that's a lesson for every age.

Alisa Harvey

DOB: September 16, 1965

Residence: Manassas, Virginia

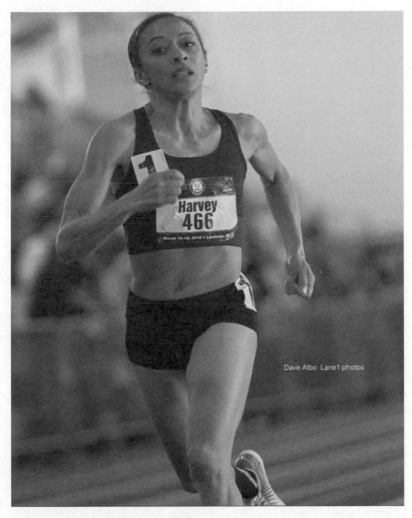

Alisa Harvey

"In it to win it."

Alisa Harvey has been competing for more than forty years, starting at age eleven. Moving through the years she has collected American indoor records in the 800 meters for age division forty, forty-five, and fifty, and world indoor 800 meters records for forty-five and fifty age groups. She also held the world indoor record for the mile in the thirty-five and forty age divisions, which has since been broken. She qualified for five Olympic trials and in 2006 Harvey was inducted into the USATF Hall of Fame. Still competing at fifty-two, she toes the line with women half her age. It used to embarrass her, but her performance is nothing to be embarrassed about. The only ones embarrassed are the twenty-year-olds who finish behind her. Married with two children, Harvey has set a high pace throughout her life.

The first thing you learn about Harvey is that she is very competitive. She says, "My nature had always been competitive. No matter if it was a game of Scrabble with my siblings or a race on the track, my goal was to figure out how to win or at least do the best that I could." She grew up in a working-class family with three siblings. Her father was a postal worker and her mother worked as a bank teller. "We weren't poor," says Harvey, "but there was always financial struggles and there was never any money to spend on extras." She played outside with her two older brothers, running after them. "I think that's where I learned to be competitive," she laughs.

In middle school, she had to participate in the Presidential Physical Fitness Test, which was administered to public school kids starting in the 1950s. Surprising herself, she did well in the 600-yard dash, beating most of the boys. Not only was she good at it, but she also loved it. She continued running for fun when she entered high school, one of five girls to run on the cross country team. She didn't know anything about form, pacing, nutrition, or gear but she found her passion. She remembers being so excited to buy her first pair of "running" shoes, which were actually light-blue tennis shoes that ended up giving her a serious case of shin splints.

In her freshman year at Thomas Jefferson High School, puberty hit and she gained weight. She saved her babysitting money to purchase vitamins and started to eat healthier. By sophomore year the weight was coming off and she hit her stride. Harvey credits her high school coach with giving her a love of competition and training. "She didn't push us too hard and really cared about us, which are good qualities in a coach," says Harvey. She finished top-five in most of her races and set the Virginia High School record for 1600 meters at 4:50, which was not broken until 2012. Harvey was determined and focused, traits that would serve her in her professional career. She describes herself as a bit of a loner, happier to spend time in the library reading up on track and field or nutrition than hanging out at a mall. Her favorite college memories aren't of prom or football games but the team trips she took to the NCAA Championships.

The summer after her senior year, before heading off college, she joined the Pinnacle Track Club where she traveled to track meets up and down the East Coast. "My running and racing progressed naturally from high school to college due to good training guidance from my coaches. I learned quickly that hard work pays of," she says.

She was offered full scholarship to five schools and selected the University of Tennessee, passing up Auburn, University of Georgia, Houston, and Florida. When asked why she chose the University of Tennessee, she explains: "My hero has always been Wilma Rudolph [the first American woman to win three gold medals in track and field at the 1960 Olympics] and I thought I had read somewhere that she went to U. of Tennessee, so that clinched the decision for me. I was so happy to be following in her footsteps. But when I got there I realized that Rudolph went to Tennessee State University!" Regardless, the choice was a good one for her. She left her mark there but it wasn't without trials and tribulations. The greatest challenge she faced in college and on the national circuit was health-related, a tendency to suffer from allergies and upper respiratory infections. "I was always prone to seasonal and indoor allergies even as a child. In high school I was able to trudge through the congestion and perform, though in college I began to develop the more serious side effects of respiratory allergies," explains Harvey. That didn't prevent her from becoming the national champion in the 1500 meter in her senior year, or being part of the Tennessee 4x800m team that set an NCAA record. She ended her college career ranked fifth in the nation in the 1500 by USATF. "I was driven to succeed, to constantly improve myself," says Harvey. "I wanted to do well for me and my family. My parents didn't get to go to college and gave me the emotional support to train hard to get here and I wanted them to be proud."

After graduating in 1987 she was picked-up by a former Nike track club, Athletics West. The club gave her a salary, performance bonuses, health insurance, and gear. For the first time in her running career she didn't have to worry about money or squeezing in her training between jobs and school work. The following year, she qualified for the Olympic trials in the 1500 but finished a disappointing eleventh place. "I wanted that so badly," she recalls. "I wanted to go to the big dance."

Shortly after that, the Athletics West Track Club dissolved. Without a team or a job, Harvey had to make one of her critical decisions in life. She moved to California and joined the Southern California Cheetahs Track Club. She also got married to her first husband and changed her name to Alisa Hill, a decision she regrets because of the confusion that it caused with her past performances and records. The move was good for her and she thrived under strong coaching and team camaraderie, competing nationally and internationally. The experience after college and stepping into the international world brought a new dimension to her training plus a raised level of competition.

Her most exciting time with the Cheetahs, and a major highlight of her career, was attending the 1991 Pan-Am Games in Havana, where she won gold in the 1500 and silver in the 800 behind Ana Quirot: "Standing on the podium was so exciting, but also it was the chance to race against Ana Quirot, the reigning world champion at 800 meters, on her home track. The crowd was so loud. Fidel Castro was in the stand cheering loudly for her." She recalls that exciting meet in detail as if it were yesterday: "There was no running hot water so my showers were cold and quick. The US Olympic Committee shipped in cases of Nutrament to help supplement the cafeteria food. We ventured into Havana and saw the hundreds of 1950s automobiles. I lounged on the beach one day between competitions. The water was as warm as bath water.

"The track stadium was not quite complete at the start of the Pan Am Games, but the track was well made and fast. I won my first event, the 1500, and got the gold medal. I remember talking to a US reporter immediately after my race. It was thrilling. I was more relaxed for my second race, the 800-meter run. There were no expectations from me as the focus was on Quirot. President Fidel Castro attended the meet to watch Quirot run.

"The 800-meter race went straight to a final, which is unusual in international competition. The rumor was that they wanted to avoid having trials in order to keep Quirot fresh for the 4x400 relay, which she would anchor. The officials lined us up on the track in lanes by groups of two. There were at least fourteen runners in the race. Quirot was positioned in her own lane up ahead of me. I was sharing one of the first two lanes. At the gun, everyone took off like it was a 400-meter sprint. After rounding the first curve I looked up to see the entire field ahead of me making a break for the inside lane. All that I could do was ride the momentum at the back of the pack. Coming into the home stretch of the first lap I was not able to challenge anyone. I just recall looking ahead and seeing everyone running single-file ahead of me. At the bell lap, I glanced at the clock to see my split read 1:00. The crowd was cheering as Quirot led the field at the bell lap. As I passed the clock I made my first move around one or two more runners while on the curve. On the backstretch I could once again see what remained of the strung-out field ahead of me. A surge of energy came on me as I made a strong surge down the backstretch. I was passing everyone. The crowd began to cheer loudly as I approached Quirot and began to challenge her. She made a quick glance over her shoulder and changed gears. The race was on. Coming around the final curve I was transfixed by Quirot's power. Her speed was far superior, but my endurance was far better. We battled into the final straightaway with the crowd coming to their feet. I kicked and sprinted as fast as I could to the line finishing second to win the silver in 1:59.99. Quirot finished just ahead of me winning the gold in 1:58.71."

While signed on with the Cheetahs, she worked at a local J. C. Penney's for income. The job was part of the Olympic Job Opportunities Program, which allowed Olympic hopefuls to work part-time and be paid full-time wages. She made extra money on the side from occasional road-race prize money earnings. "The demand on time was great as there are only twenty-four hours in a day and time management is key," as Harvey would soon learn. Her first marriage in 1990 was a good decision at the time. "The stability of owning a condo, going to work, and training daily with my club teammates was a positive for me," she explains. "I had some of my best career performances during the early nineties." Then she made another decision that would affect her career. She got pregnant and gained sixty pounds. The prize was the birth of her daughter, Virginia Hill, in 1994. "In that era most people did not expect me to return to track. After I had lost the baby weight and resumed competing, I was on a flight with the former American record holder in the mile, Steve Scott. He asked me why I had decided to have a child right in the middle of my career. I didn't have an eloquent response to Scott's question. I simply wanted to have a baby while I was in my late twenties."

When recounting the decades, Harvey sees her twenties as one of her best running decades. She blossomed and was focused and relentless on the track. But her early thirties were tumultuous. It started out with a typical Harvey bang, winning the 1999 Fifth Avenue Mile in 4:29:65 and then qualifying for the US Olympic Trials marathon in 2000, "a total fluke!" She never planned to run a marathon and then place second in her first attempt. "It was one of my accomplishments that brought me much pride and satisfaction," she recalls. But then her marriage started to deteriorate. She was left with little childcare to train and no assistance from her husband. She took the baby to the Kentucky Derby Mile, and the race director provided childcare for her. At thirty-two her marriage dissolved. She worked two jobs and tried to make some cash at road races at any distance running the mile to the ten-mile and everything in between. She started coaching herself, training with a baby jogger. She ran road races on the weekends when family could watch the baby. "I was determined and hungry to succeed," says Harvey. As much as she loved being a mother, training and racing became instantly more difficult.

She made another life-changing decision in 2001 and remarried, having her second child, a son, in 2002. That brought her the emotional support and financial stability she needed to continue her professional running. "My more mature self made a better relationship decision the second time around, and I found the right guy!" She came back to training and competing with a vengeance. She was coaching at George Mason University and did all the workouts with the college kids. "That really boosted my training," she laughs. "I worked as hard as they did!" As well as she was running, Harvey noticed a slight decrease in her speed by her mid-forties. "Everything just got a little harder," she says. "Then on top of aging, factor in all the hormone changes!" Despite all that, she broke indoor masters' mile record with a time of 4:48.

Her fifth decade, now in the masters division, started out with a win at the Army Ten-Miler and setting a masters American indoor mile record. She finds her sixth decade liberating. Still competing, she has tightened her range of races, swearing off marathons. "That's a younger person's distance," she laughs. "Too hard on the body." Stretching, massage, and foam-rolling and other tools are now part of her regular maintenance routine. Adequate rest and recovery are also key components in her regime, as is managing injuries. "If I feel something uncomfortable in my muscles or joints, I stop the workout immediately," says Harvey. She regularly uses a recumbent cycle and installed a pull-up bar and weights in her house. She still takes those multivitamins she started taking as a kid. "Historically, my running has gone downhill every time I lose my mind and get caught up with some ridiculous nutrition plan," says Harvey. "As I get older it isn't easy to continue to push myself physically or mentally. Since I have been training at a high level for so many years, it gets harder to motivate myself to hurt. But I am hopelessly competitive. Competition is a motivator for me. I will hurt for the chance to win."

She talks about other aging factors such as her heart rate. She's been using a heart rate monitor throughout her career and has recorded the information. The changes as she ages are noteworthy: "My maximum heart rate at fifty is 193. When I was in my twenties, it was 222. Unfortunately, I'm always trying to compare my younger self to my now older self." Her older self is doing quite well. She broke the World 50 world indoor record for 800 meters and the following weekend broke her own record. She describes her routine: "I use races as training for other races. My ten-mile races help train me for my 5K and 10K races. My 5K and 10K road races help train me for my 1500 and mile races. My 1500 and mile races help train me for my 800-meter races. The reverse works as well. I believe the true key to my success is that I have been able to use my natural speed to make my longer races more efficient."

George Banker has been mentoring Harvey since she came on the DC racing scene. He shared his interviews on Harvey with me as part of my research on her and they are a contributing factor to this profile. Banker describes Harvey at the track: "While running around the track you can see the intensity in her eyes. Each step that is taken around the track is with determination. She floats around the track effortlessly."

Another aging lesson this world-class competitor has learned is to be social while running. She enjoys running turkey trots with her kids and savoring the time with them. She has a circle of running friends that she runs with at any pace, enjoying the camaraderie. But when the competitive juices kick in, there's no stopping her. At a Turkey Trot 5K she ran a 19:19 at age fifty-two. When she lines up at races against college runners, which she sometimes does as part of her George Mason coaching, she says the women initially look at her as if to say, "What are you doing here old lady?" But when the gun goes off and the elbows start flying, she holds her own. "They force me to run harder and I like that," she laughs. At one of these recent races she took second place against the college women and said, "It probably isn't any fun for them finishing behind a fifty-two-year-old woman!"

With thirty years of elite running behind her and still in the game in her fifties, Harvey is in a place to look back on her career but also look forward. What she has learned is that it isn't always about winning but putting forth the maximum effort. The future holds excitement for her, as she sees no limit to her goals. "Running has enhanced my life so much. The friendships, the travel, and the reach of knowing I did my best," says Harvey.

Another passion she found through running is a love of nature and gardening. As a city girl who grew up in a trailer, she now loves being outdoors and has developed a deep connection to nature. She relishes time in her garden surrounded by sunflowers and hydrangeas, which she finds relaxing and almost meditative. Calming affects this super-competitive woman needs.

Harvey's life has not been easy but to talk to her one would never know the struggles. She laughs a lot, is proud of her kids—her daughter competed in the 400-meter-hurdles at college and her son wrestles— and she is totally in love with her husband, "the right one." She's handled her disappointments in life like those on the track, with candor and objectivity: "I review the facts, come to a logical reason for what happened and I just move on." Her future goals are without limits. She looks up to world record senior competitors in their late sixties, such as Kathy Martin and Sabra Harvey, and hopes to achieve what they have. Summing up her life and career, Harvey eloquently states: "My love of staying fit and being competitive is what keeps my fire burning on the roads and on the track." Her fire will burn bright for many years.

Sabra Harvey

DOB: March 2, 1949

Residence: Houston, Texas

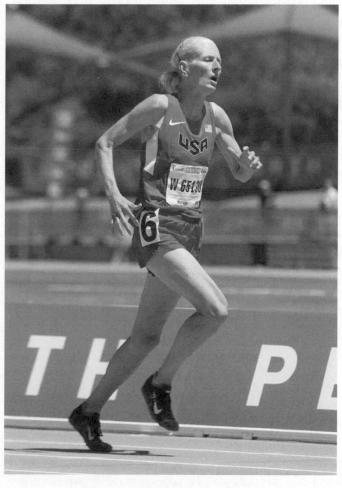

Sabra Harvey

"I'm enjoying the journey."

Don't underestimate Sabra Harvey on any level. She is a formidable competitor and trains like a warrior. She came late to running, picking up the sport at fifty-one at the suggestion of a co-worker. Her first event was a 50K trail walk, followed by a road 5K, and she fell in love with the sport and with competition. She's worked with a coach and is now one of the top female masters runners in the country. Harvey is having the time of her life and has learned to balance her family with her training and still have time to babysit grandchildren on occasion.

"If you had told me at age fifty that within a few years I would morph into a hard-driving, competitive runner, I would have laughed," says Harvey, who never ran or did any sports as a child. She grew up on a farm in south Texas and spent a lot of time playing outdoors. She didn't play organized sports, preferring time spent with the local 4-H chapter, taking care of animals. "I had no desire for cheerleading or flag twirling or other extracurricular activities that passed as girls' sports back then," she affirms loud and clear. At home she did household chores such as feeding the horses and doing the dishes after meals. Saturday mornings she and her three sisters were expected to clean the house before watching cartoons or going outside, but they figured out a way to sneak out some days without doing the chores. She walked a half-mile to the bus stop in first grade on a dirt path along a canal. She gets upset when she hears that parents today don't allow their kids to walk to school or a bus stop even if it is close by. "Kids have no independence today," she says. "And that is something missing in their life experiences."

By the end of high school, she had outgrown small-town life and attended college first in North Texas and then in New Mexico. She graduated with degrees in secondary education and art. Her career took a back seat to marriage and two sons. She shared her love of the outdoors with the boys, spending time camping, hiking, skiing, and fishing. She coached one of her sons' soccer team. Life went by at a steady pace in Los Alamos. Before she knew it, she was fifty.

A move to Houston in 1996 was followed in four years by another move to the Washington, DC, area. With the boys established in school, she took a job as a graphic designer spending her days behind a desk. "I was up to 160 pounds and actually not really aware of being there," she recalls. "I was challenged to hike (i.e. walk) a mountainous 50K and thought, *well I can walk that far—it's only walking*! It was never about losing weight or getting fit. I thought I was both fit and skinny anyway having been that way all of my life!" It was only several years later after seeing a photo of herself that she realized she was not so "mean and lean." She started walking with friends at work, and prodded on by one of them, the group signed up for the Dogwood Half Hundred, a 50K endurance hike through Virginia's George Washington National Forest. For Harvey, it was like being a kid again. She loved the long days in the mountains and socializing with her teammates. When they finished the walk, the woman who organized them said, "For our next event we are tackling a 5K." Harvey's reaction? "You've got to be kidding," she recalls at the thought of running 3.1 miles.

But she threw her hat in and trained at a local track. "Once around the track was enough for me," she laughs. On race day, though, caught up by the excitement of the race and the exhilaration of competition, she sprinted to the finish. Surprised at her own reaction, Harvey examined her nature: "I thought I was more the laidback type but eventually came to own up to my competitive nature," she says. "I'm very competitive!"

She started running on weekends, just for the fun of it. She signed up for local races but didn't take herself seriously. "I didn't know about running shoes, clothing, pace, or any aspect of training," she recalls. When her husband changed jobs back to Houston, she decided to become more of a runner and searched for a beginner's running club in her new hometown. She signed up for a ten-week beginner's clinic and formed a friendly relationship with one of the coaches, Karen Bowler, who ran with the Houston Striders. Bowler immediately saw the hidden potential in Harvey and started to work with Harvey one-on-one. "She convinced me I could run faster and win my age group," says Harvey. "She had a knack for seeing things in me that I didn't. She brought out the best in me."

Under Bowler's watchful eye, Harvey's times started to drop. Her 5K time went from 24:00 to under 20:00. At age sixty, she PRed with a 19:12. When asked what the magic was, how Bowler got her to those times, Harvey doesn't have much of a magical response. "I worked hard because Karen believed in me. She kept telling me I had the talent, that it was there, I just needed to tap into it," said Harvey. "She let me discover myself and kept my mental attitude positive when I had self-doubts."

In 2016 Harvey went to Perth, Australia to participate in the World Masters Athletics Championships. She worked with Bowler via

email—she had moved to the UK—on a twelve-week plan. Her ultimate goal was to set a world record for 800 meters. She'd come close
to setting it two years prior, and the near miss stuck in her craw. Bowler's training philosophy for the WMAs was to keep things simple. She
told Harvey not to over-train, over-stress, or make things complicated.
Bowler told her to finish every workout tired but with enough left that
she could do more. "I was never gobsmacked by the training," Harvey
affirms. It worked. At the Games, she set an age-group world record of
2:39 for 800 meters, placed second in the 5000 meters in 20:40, and
won gold in the 1500 meters in 5:39. "Sometimes it's hard for me to
believe I did that!" says Harvey in her signature dry tone. Tall and lean,
she can be hard to read, which drives her competitors crazy. Her expres-
sion has been described as unfriendly, a bit hard. She's been told to smile
more. But beneath that she has a humorous side and a dry wit. She likes
to laugh at herself and never takes her accomplishments for granted. If
you saw her at a party you might not engage with her at first, but that
would be a mistake. Harvey runs deep.

During her years of aggressive training and racing she has only
suffered one major injury. Six years ago she fell while running in a relay
and shattered her right shoulder. It took a year for her to heal from the
surgery. "I could feel it happen," she recalls. "I was running too fast and
didn't hydrate properly during the five miles and the legs just gave out."
Other than that, "I've just had my fair share of niggles."

When asked about coming late to the game, Harvey has a well-
thought-out and reflective response: "Timing is everything," she says.
"If I had started younger, I probably wouldn't have been as focused as I
am now." She believes in the old adage that things in life happen when
they are supposed to happen. She reflects on how her life has changed
since she became a world-class runner. During her training season, her
day starts with a run. It took her husband and sons a few years to accept
her routine and vigorous training schedule. Throw in all the travel to
races she needed to attend, both national and international, and they
were looking at a new woman.

"My family is still my priority, but sometimes I have to say no to
babysitting!" she laughs. "Now my son asks me well in advance and is
hesitant to ask me during my racing season." Her husband used to attend her races at the beginning of her career to make sure she was safe,
but now he stays home most of the time. "My family are my team and

they are very supportive," says Harvey. "When they came to accept that this is the path I was pursuing and that I was serious and committed, they were on board."

Her team also consists of Coach Karen on an as-needed basis, and Harvey sees a chiropractor every few weeks for soft tissue work to knead out the knots. She's also tweaked her diet. She has eliminated milk, cut down some on meat, and added more fruit and fish. In her off-season, November through January, she takes a breather from the intensity and runs just for herself, "just for the fun of it."

Like most competitors on the masters' circuit, Harvey has made friends with other runners. Another highly competitive runner, Kathy Martin, often runs against Harvey. "We are friendly competitors," says Harvey of her age-group nemesis. They stand toe-to-toe on the start line. "I'd rather see her next to me than wonder where she is behind me and when she's going to make a move," explains Harvey. "We have different tactics and I stick to my own plan." Sticking to her plan has worked well for Harvey. Over the years of tough competition, she has become more confident. She is learning when to make her move and has edged out Martin a few times recently. Part of the skill and strategy of competition is knowing what you are good at and sticking to it. Harvey feels she is better suited to the middle distances on the track and shorter road events (up to ten miles). This is her sweet spot.

In January 2017, she gave some thought to her annual goals. She's considering going for the age-group world record for 5000 meters on the track. To do that she'll need to run below 20:08. In researching the current record, she wasn't surprised to see that Kathy Martin set the world 5K road record of 19:57 in October of 2016. The bar just got higher if she wants to go for that as well. In July of 2017, she will compete at the USATF Masters Outdoor Championships in Baton Rouge, aiming for a record in the road 5K. Coming from Texas, the heat won't be a factor; in fact it could be an advantage against runners from cooler climates.

During training season that starts in February, Harvey is up at 5:30 a.m. to beat the heat. She'll eat half a banana with peanut butter and then head out to meet her training partner. Depending on the schedule, sometimes they'll do an easy run, while at other times they pick up the pace and do drills. Her partner is a marathoner, which actually works out well. "We talk a lot when we aren't doing drills," says Harvey. "I love the company." Harvey has encouraged her partner to come to the masters' meet in Baton Rouge and even though there isn't a marathon event, her partner is psyched to enter her first masters track-and-field event. "That's just one of the benefits of having a running buddy," says Harvey. "We encourage each other to try out new things."

When I next catch up with Harvey, it is October of 2017. I want to find out how she did in Baton Rouge at the USATF Masters Outdoor Championships. Ever humble, she says she did well. I have to ask a few more questions before she tells me she placed first in all her events; the 800, 1500, and 5000 meters. After the meet she took a recovery week, which means she still ran but at a low intensity. One month later, she was in Michigan for the Bobby Crim one-mile and ten-mile events, placing first in her age division with times of 6:07 and 1:11:55, respectively. A month later she planned to break that 5K road record at the Syracuse Masters 5K Championships, but a larger-than-life force put her training on hold—Hurricane Harvey.

The hurricane hit Houston as she and her training partner, Lynn Malloy, were running the Crim 10 Mile. Afterward, she dashed to the airport—but all flights to Houston were already cancelled. They were able to get a flight to Dallas and then drove the four hours to Houston, "one step ahead of the storm surge," she recalls. The next day she and her husband Bill had to evacuate and they had minutes to grab their essentials. "I grabbed my running shoes and my running bras," Harvey said. "I lost all my running medals, articles, photos, and books." With her dry sense of humor, she laughs that at least now she won't have to figure what to keep and what to throw away, since it's all gone.

She and her husband lost everything. For the first three weeks after the storm, they lived with her son and then were able to park a travel trailer in their driveway of their house. The sixteen-foot trailer barely has room for Harvey and her husband, their two dogs, a small sleeping area and a stove for basically making coffee. The house had to be gutted down to the studs. Between the hurricane, the devastation of her home and now living out of a trailer, her training for Syracuse was put on hold. She tried training the morning after the hurricane subsided but couldn't find any dry land. It took a week for her to find dry spots like a golf course and three weeks before she could run her usual route in a park. Her preparation for the 5K record was not ideal and she had no illusions that she would break it. She ran a 20:44, needing to go under 19:57. It was frustrating for her as she ran a 19:51 during a training run.

But with her no-nonsense attitude, she says she'll "just reset that one and try again."

Harvey thinks about the path her life has taken. "Mine is an interesting life for sure," she says. Growing up in the pre–Title IX era, she was not allowed to join a track team in school, didn't have any female role models. She is learning about the female pioneers in our sport and is grateful for their determination. When she started competing in 2004, she was shocked at some of the male chauvinism she encountered. "At the start line I would hear men say, 'I'm not letting that woman beat me,'" she recalls. "It made me so mad that I was determined to leave them in my dust, and I did." She recalls running with two men at a local club and at the end of the session she suggested they do a cool down. Instead of cooling down, they sped up to beat her. "I thought, *What dummies*," she laughs. "This was a cool down, but they wanted to be the peacocks. So I sprinted by them really fast and then waited for them at the end. They both came over to me very humbled and said they'd never do that again!" She's not so much a feminist as she is concerned about being respectful. "As runners, we should be helping each other," she says. "Except at a race when the stakes are high and everyone is on their own." But even then, she'll be the first to congratulate the winner and cheer for everyone.

Harvey ended 2017 with a bang. In October, she was selected as the USA Track and Field's Masters Athlete of the Year. She traveled to Ohio for her award and was humbled at the experience: "Being selected Master Athlete of the Year is quite an honor. I was gobsmacked. It is recognition of a body of work this year that could not have been much better. I just had a goal and was building to get there. Realizing how many worthy athletes could or were considered for the honor, I was just taken aback at being plucked from a crowded field of elite athletes. Also, pretty heady stuff receiving the award in Ohio and 'rubbing elbows' with the likes of Emma Coburn and Dan O'Brien." Harvey is not one to rest on her laurels. The Saturday after her award presentation, she took another age-graded win at the 6K cross-country nationals in Lexington, Kentucky, in 26:15.

Summing up her newfound life, Harvey reflects: "Running makes me feel independent, free, strong, and confident. I've managed to fit running into my life at a time when I could pursue it and I find it to be so fulfilling. I'm enjoying the journey and feel like a very lucky woman."

Julia Hawkins

DOB: February 10, 1916

Residence: Baton Rouge, Louisiana

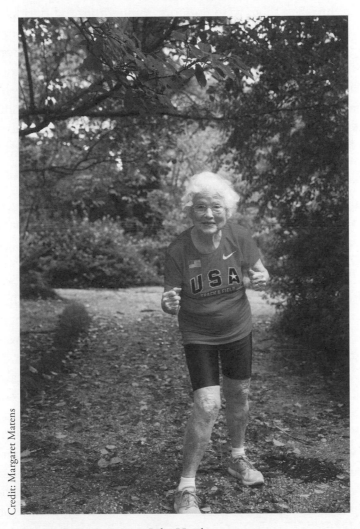

Credit: Margaret Matens

Julia Hawkins

"It's never too late."

Julia Hawkins started running at a hundred. At the 2017 National Senior Olympic Games in Birmingham, Alabama, she ran the 100-yard dash in 39.62, setting a world record in the age group. The following month at the USATF Outdoor championship in Baton Rouge, she ran it again in 40.12 proving she wasn't a one-hit wonder. Already a gold medalist in the National Senior Games for cycling—she was a fixture at the National Senior Games starting in 1995 and accrued three gold medals in the 5K and 10K time trials in cycling at age eighty—she stopped competing in that event when there were no more competitors and decided to run instead. "I don't feel 102," she states. "More like sixty or seventy. But nothing, especially age, is going to stop me from doing what I want."

When I call Julia she is outside attending to the bonsai plants in the yard that she has been nurturing for forty years. Baton Rouge is having a cold snap, the temperature dropped down to 20 degrees Fahrenheit, and she needs to make sure the roots are kept warm. She hauls around a five-pound hose to water them every day and laughs that this is her weight strengthening exercise. "I'm always doing yard work and running for the phone," she explains. "This is how I stay in shape."

Julia Hawkins was born in Delevan, Wisconsin, however a few months afterwards her family moved to Ponchatoula, Louisiana. Hawkins's mind is sharp as a tack and she recalls scenes from her childhood with vivid memory. Soon after her parents settled, her mother opened a tea room and served tea, homemade pies, and fried oyster po'boys. The success of the tea room led to managing a hotel and finally the family bought a beach hotel in Ponchatoula that they ran as a summer resort. Hawkins was given lots of chores to do, but when her sister was born, she was put in charge of her as a "little mother." In her memoir, *It's Been Wondrous*, she recalls putting the baby in her bike basket and taking her for a ride. Hawkins was a pretty little girl with long blonde curls but she was also a tomboy, mischievous and a talker. She was once paid five cents to just sit still and be quiet for five minutes.

She attended school in town, a six-mile bus ride. After being dropped off at home after school, she never made it back for extracurricular activities or sports, which she regrets. When the Depression hit, things got tough and the family had to watch every penny. She and her family picked strawberries in the early spring to earn extra money. At the hotel, they rationed provisions to make sure the guests ate well.

Hawkins recalls eating chicken necks because "the good parts had to be saved for the guests." Her mother sewed all her clothes and mended her stockings. Despite the hardships, she looks back on her childhood fondly. For a child, living at the beach was magical. She recalls bonfires, starry nights, and boat rides, but also the hard work of running a summer hotel such as preparing over one hundred chicken dinners every night, which entailed "killing the chickens, plucking them, cutting them up, and frying them."

In her senior year of high school the family moved to Baton Rouge where her two older brothers were attending Louisiana State University (LSU) and where she would soon follow. That is where she met the love of her life. On the first day of school at LSU, Julia met Buddy Hawkins at an Episcopal Student Center mixer and "lost her heart" to the tall blonde who would become her future husband. She was a good student and managed to get in her studies while working all kinds of jobs to help offset the cost of college. Her work ethic was boundless, a trait she would carry with her throughout life and on to the masters games.

She graduated with a teaching degree and bought a Model-A Ford to commute to work, teaching fourth grade. Although she was keen to be married, Buddy wasn't, at least not yet; not one to sit around, Hawkins applied for a teaching job with the United Fruit Company at a banana plantation in Honduras and spent a year teaching the children of the employees. This was in 1938. You have to admire her pluckiness to travel so far alone. Hawkins loved the travel, the excitement and newness of the journey. Being open to new possibilities seems to be a trait Hawkins always had and used to its full advantage. When she returned home at the end of the year, she brought back a monkey—bad idea—and a collection of exotic orchids—good idea—that thrived in the Louisiana climate.

Returning from Honduras in late 1938, Julia and Buddy renewed their relationship and love but World War II was looming and Buddy was sent to Pearl Harbor. When the attack happened on December 7, 1941, it wasn't until eight painful days later that she finally heard from him. He was being shipped out right away and proposed over the phone. She of course said yes, but then came the surprise part. They were to be married over the phone as well since there was no time for Julia to get to Hawaii before he left port. It took months of letter writing, finding pastors who would perform the unusual ceremony, and getting loved ones together before they could go forward with the marriage. On November 29, 1942, at the Ponchatoula Savings and Loan Office on one side and the US Navy on the other, Julia and Buddy were married over the phone. As Hawkins recalls: "It was a bit of a lonely wedding night . . . but I was happy knowing we legally belonged to each other." As a wedding present she bought herself a bike to commute to school. The war rationing of gasoline made it impossible to drive her Model-A. Years later, for their fiftieth wedding anniversary, their four children and grandchildren gave them a party complete with a three-tiered wedding cake and wedding veil for Julia.

After the war, Buddy received his teaching degree and taught at LSU until he retired in 1977 as head of the petroleum engineering department. The couple settled down in Baton Rouge, eventually raising their kids. Buddy built their house and most of the furniture in it. Ever resourceful and cost-efficient, Julia kept the Model-A Ford because "it still ran and wasn't quite an antique just yet." Their first dog, a fox terrier, would sit on the running board while she drove the car.

After all the hard work and toil that Julia put in from an early age, she didn't need sports. She was active every day. She rode her bike to work. She gardened. She loved to swim and paddle boats on the lake. She was a baseball coach at one of the schools where she taught. She took her students on field trips. She loved to hike. She tried going to exercise classes but other things, like a fishing trip, got in the way. When she and Buddy retired at age seventy, they took up biking, averaging one thousand miles a year. For her seventieth birthday, she received a Schwinn bike with a speedometer so she could see how far and how fast she went around the neighborhood. Her lifestyle was active and healthy, which paved the way for her to start competing at one hundred.

She's been writing her life story since she was fifty and as a one-hundredth birthday present, her kids had her memoirs published. Julia tells me to buy her book so I don't have to interview her but speaking with her is so much fun I keep the interview going. And then I order the book.

In 1994, at age seventy-eight, she was encouraged by her younger sister Mickey to enter the Louisiana Senior Games. Hawkins entered the 5K and one-mile bike event, taking home two gold medals. She recalls that day: "When my turn came, I zipped off and found it great fun and quite a challenge. There was no one in my age group, but my times were better than the ladies in the next younger group, so I felt pretty good."

Her next competition was the National Senior Olympics in San Antonio, Texas in 1995. She questioned the need for going, wondering why, at her age, she was starting to compete. "Why do I do it? Do I need a challenge? My life is good, why do I want to add strain to it?" But since her children and Buddy were very supportive and enthusiastic, she decided to enter the 5K and one-mile bike event. She practiced every day, riding her bike through the neighborhood. The day before the race she did a trial run on the 5K course and was alarmed to find it very hilly and her five-speed bike not sufficient to climb the hills. A frantic call was put into a local bike shop and the owner came up with a ten-speed bike he thought she could handle. Said Hawkins of learning gears on a bike the day before her race: "This business of teaching old dogs new tricks wasn't too easy!" The day of the race she recalls saying: "What have I gotten myself into? Everyone needs a challenge but not this far and not this much!" She placed fifth in the 5K and took bronze in the one-mile and was thrilled. "After all, I was at the end of the age group!" she laughs. Hawkins competed four more times at the National Games in the bike events, getting gold in the 5K and 10K three out of the four times. At the National Senior Games in 1977 in Tucson, Arizona, she won gold in the 5K and 10K bike event on the same day. As she recalls it, she sounds like a teenager: "I felt like I was flying as I passed the three that started before me. I was so high it took awhile to come down. The adrenaline was flowing." She stopped competing when there was no one to compete against in her age group. "The women just drop off after a certain age," she stated.

In 1997, she was featured in an article in *Sports Illustrated* for her Nationals biking events. They traveled all over the globe together, sometimes with the kids and grandkids. For her ninety-fifth birthday in 2012, she and Buddy put on a Mardi Gras bike parade with one hundred friends in costume complete with Mardi Gras beads. They decorated their bikes and rode through town. She still rode her bike every day. But soon Buddy started to fail and by March of 2013 was suffering poor health. Julia recalls the night he died: "We lay in bed together, and he sang me love songs which he would do." He died peacefully in his sleep after seventy years of marriage. In her memoir, Hawkins shares some of his love letters to her over the years. They are tender and filled with love.

At ninety-eight, she fell off her bike and dislocated her right elbow. The pain was awful and she felt helpless. She spent her recovery watching

LSU football games. And as soon as the cast came off, she was back on her bike. For her ninety-ninth birthday, the theme of the party was "A charmed life." Her kids gave her a necklace and then for the remainder of the weekend, Hawkins was put on a treasure hunt to find the charms. It was pretty easy to figure out what the charms would be: a Model-A, an LSU tiger, a bike, and a telephone representing her marriage, among others.

For her one-hundredth birthday, she was feted with bands, a parade, and a roomful of 250 guests at a banquet hall at Louisiana State University. The surprise guest was the LSU Tiger. Prior to the big event on her actual birthday, she was given small smatterings of celebrations for the one hundred days leading up to February 10. Photos of the birthday bash prove Hawkins is vibrant, kicking up her dance steps to the New Orleans jazz band that played at the party. She is the epitome of a woman who has lived a charmed life and isn't ready to relinquish one moment of it.

At one hundred, Hawkins picked up a new sport—running. Setting her sites on the National Senior Olympics in June of 2016, she started practicing. One of her sons marked off a 50-meter stretch in her yard so she could practice when she felt like it. She qualified for the Nationals at the Louisiana State Games in Lake Charles with ease, winning gold in the 50-meter. When it came time for the Nationals in Birmingham, Alabama, she added the 100-meter dash because, "Well, I'm one hundred so why not run the 100?!" And Hawkins discovered she loved running for the same reasons young people pick up the sport. "It gave me a sense of freedom. It lets me be independent," she explains. "With running, it's just me and my body. I can just go out and do the best I can and not depend on anything else."

At the National Senior Olympics in June of 2017 at age 101, Hawkins set an age group world record for the 100-yard dash in 39.62. Her accomplishment went viral and she was dubbed "Hurricane Hawkins." Her daughter had to teach her to Google her name so we could see all the articles written about her from the *Washington Post*, *Runners World*, and the local papers. A month later she ran the 100-yard dash at the USA Track & Field Masters Outdoor Championships in her hometown of Baton Rouge, clocking a 40.12. "I wanted to beat my world record, but I was happy with that," states Hawkins.

Of all the events she entered, the outdoor championships at the LSU field, brought back many memories. "Standing at the start, I looked out across the field and could see the place where Buddy's dorm had been. It's now the football stadium. And I could see where I lived, which is now the Field House. The view brought back so many wonderful memories of my life with Buddy and our fabulous years at LSU," says Hawkins.

Her fifteen minutes of fame lasted for months. She's been on NBC, CBS, NPR, Fox News, and other media outlets. Everywhere she went people wanted their picture taken with her. "I must have had my photo taken one thousand times," she laughs. She's been invited to speak at Rotary clubs and retirement homes and was invited to a Saints Football Game where she was introduced on the field.

Hawkins has a lot to say about turning 102 (although she states she feels sixty) and being fit, active, and inspiring. Here are just a few of her tips:

1. Keep moving. Whether it's gardening, housework, or walking, be active.
2. There is a fine line between pushing yourself and wearing yourself out. Don't overdo it; just be the best you can be. When I compete, I want to spend all my energy on the track but have a little bit left to wave to my family and friends at the finish.
3. Don't worry about things you can't control. At 101, anything could happen. But I don't worry about that.
4. Surround yourself with family and friends. They are the most important things in life. Be a part of a community.
5. Enjoy everyday "Magic Moments" that take your breath away. Maybe it's a flower in bloom or a sunset. Notice and appreciate the natural world around us.

George Hirsch

DOB: June 21, 1934

Residence: Manhattan, New York

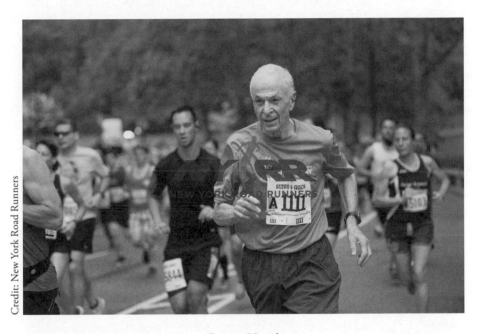

George Hirsch

"How did I get so lucky?"

George Aaron Hirsch has led many lives. He is a marathoner (forty of them), Princeton and Harvard educated, a one-time candidate for US Congress, and by all counts a Renaissance man. At eighty-four, he can place in his age at a 10K, go home and cook up a delicious Italian meal paired with the best Chianti, and serve it to a number of running friends who always stop by to say hello. He might then fly anywhere around the world to collect honors and accolades for his lifetime achievements which are many, starting with running a 3:31 marathon at age seventy-one and a 2:03 half-marathon at eighty. Engaging, kind, and always with a ready smile, Hirsch makes aging look easy. There are many things Hirsch is passionate about, but his wife Shay, who passed away in 2014, will always be number one for him.

His running history is legendary. In 1976, at age thirty-two, he ran the first New York City Marathon in 2 hours and 49 minutes. At age fifty, he ran it in 3 hours and 3 minutes. His most infamous marathons were the back-to-back Chicago/New York City in 2009. Hirsch, then seventy-five, ran the Chicago Marathon in 3 hours and 58 minutes as a warm-up to New York. One month later when he crossed the finish line of the New York City Marathon in a time of 4 hours and 6 minutes, he placed first in his age division. But he didn't feel great and the race took its toll. Despite a little help from his friends Amby Burfoot, Bill Rodgers, and Germán Silva, all of whom met Hirsch along the course for emotional support, he felt wobbly. He thought he might collapse. By the time he finished, all he wanted was to find his wife Shay and go for coffee and cheesecake. Shay was not happy with his condition and made him promise that it would be his last marathon. After forty marathons with a PR of 2:38 in the 1979 Boston Marathon, he was ready to relinquish his marathon days. He made the promise and kept it.

"I was never a good runner in high school. I joined the team because I loved sports but wasn't very talented, so I needed a team where I wouldn't be cut," says Hirsch of his humble beginnings as a runner. He continued running at Princeton but was a mediocre athlete. After college, he joined the Navy for three years and was stationed in Naples, Italy (hence his passion for Italian food). Running took a back seat, but he did join the Running of the Bulls at Pamplona, in which, he says, he wasn't very courageous. "I ran so fast I never saw a bull," he recalls.

In 1967, after a career at Time Inc., he began to publish a start-up called *New York* magazine. It launched in April of 1968. "That was an incredible time in our country," he recalls. "The first week of publication, Martin Luther King Jr. was assassinated. That was followed with Bobby Kennedy's assassination six weeks later and the riots in Chicago that summer during the Democratic National Convention." The staff writers included Gloria Steinem and Tom Wolfe. Hirsch worked day and night on his magazine, with no time for any exercise, and he got out of shape. "The belt buckle was definitely getting tight," he laughs. He started to run to get fitter but didn't know quite how to go about it. He recalls putting on a big clunky stopwatch and running around the block as fast as he could. His only plan was to run faster every time he went out.

In 1968, running as a sport or hobby was still in its infancy. There weren't many books on the subject for Hirsch to read. During a run one day he saw another runner and they stopped to talk. The runner was Vince Chiappetta, then president of NYRR, who along with Fred Lebow would organize the first New York City Marathon in 1970. Chiappetta took Hirsch under his wing: he taught him about road running and introduced him to living legends like George Sheehan and Ted Corbitt. To Hirsch, Chiappetta was a godsend, and he soaked up his vast running knowledge. Under his guidance, Hirsch ramped up the miles and the speed, and he loved it. Feeling ready to go the distance, he entered the 1969 Boston Marathon. "I sent in my two-dollar entry fee and a letter from a doctor saying I was fit to run," he recalls. He wrote to Andy Crichton and Walt Bingham, writers for *Sports Illustrated* at the time, for advice. According to Hirsch, their advice was as follows: "Eat a big breakfast that includes a stack of pancakes, a bowl of oatmeal, an English muffin, and a glass of orange juice. Drive to Hopkinton [there were no buses to the start back then] on Route 128—do not drive the course or you will not want to run back." Hirsch still has the letter.

He recalls his first Boston Marathon: "I was standing on the start line with George Sheehan, who introduced me to all his friends as his protégé. I hadn't run over twenty miles in training, so I was apprehensive. When I crested Heartbreak Hill, there was a policeman with a megaphone who yelled out to all the runners, 'Your achievement is superb! Only six miles to go.' At that point, I knew I would finish. Tears came to my eyes." His time was 3:26, and like many exhausted first-timers, he claimed he would never run another marathon. "Too long, too hard, too much wear and tear on the body," he said. But soon after he recovered, he started planning his next one.

Back in New York, Hirsch attended a dinner party with the television host David Susskind. Hirsch casually mentioned that he'd just run the Boston Marathon, and everyone became intrigued. Running a marathon, especially Boston, was so far off the radar back then that Susskind decided to make it the headliner of his next show. A week later, Hirsch found himself on television with Sheehan, Chiappetta, and Crichton discussing the marathon. A new chapter in his life was just beginning, one that would have running at its core.

Hirsch became ensconced in the New York City and Boston Marathon scene. He helped Fred Lebow move the Marathon from the confines of Central Park out to the five boroughs in 1976 to celebrate the nation's bicentennial. In 1979, Hirsch founded the Midnight Run in New York's Central Park. From 1984 to 1986, he was the on-air host of a weekly segment on ESPN's *SportsCenter*. He did television commentary for running events including the New York City, Boston, Los Angeles, San Francisco, and Cincinnati Marathons. He's been a commentator for three Olympic Games: Los Angeles in 1984, Seoul in 1988, and Barcelona in 1992. He is still a sought-after encyclopedia on all things related to the marathon. Most runners will know him as the worldwide publisher of *Runner's World* from 1987 to 2004.

Despite his Ivy League pedigree and publishing career mingling with celebrities, Hirsch does not put on airs. He is just the opposite. When we meet, it's usually at some local coffee shop where he greets all the staff by name. When he walks into the offices at NYRR, it's more of an ambling gait than an aristocratic walk, clutching a dog-eared brief-case in hand that holds the *New York Times* and other reading material. He stops at everyone's desk to chat and inquire about their families. If a new employee walks by, he introduces himself. He takes the A train when commuting from his home in Harlem. He likes to schmooze and to have fun. He truly is the "Chairman of the Board of Running," respected and admired by many.

Hirsch is a man of conviction, determination, and passion. The best example of his determination is the story of how he met his wife, Shay. He was attending the 1988 Olympic Marathon Trials, which were being held at the New Jersey Waterfront Marathon. He was in the *Runner's World* expo booth when he caught sight of a pretty woman who was there to run her first marathon. They made eye contact and Hirsch felt smitten from the start. She moved on. Hirsch followed her and introduced himself. They struck up a conversation about her marathon and he asked her what her goal was. "Just to finish," she said. And then added, "but I'd like to qualify for Boston." Hirsch asked her out for dinner, but she declined. The next morning Hirsch stood at the start line scanning the crowds for Shay. He was dressed to run even though he hadn't run a marathon in five years. When the last runners passed, he started at the back of the pack and worked his way through the crowd until he found her at the five-mile mark. She was surprised to see him and when asked what he was doing there he replied, "I'm looking for you."

He talked to her the entire way and they found they had much in common. At the finish, Hirsch stepped aside, and Shay crossed in 3:37, her BQ time. They were married a year later in Central Park. Shay and George were rarely apart for the next twenty-five years until she passed away in 2014 after a long battle with cancer.

At eighty-four, Hirsch is not ready to retire or stop running. Why should he? He leads an active life that would leave many half his age suffering from sleep deprivation. He has kept his promise to his late wife not to compete in any more marathons, but he still runs, and well. "The competitive feeling is still alive and kicking," he proclaimed. When running in New York, his main competitor is Witold Bialokur. "He's the star. I can't beat him," says Hirsch. "But that doesn't mean I don't try!" His running form has never been fluid, more of a slouch, and he now has to be careful not to fall. A friend described his form: "He doesn't glide over the road; he moves ahead in a determined shuffle. He runs with his heart and his steel-tough mind, telling his skinny legs, cramp-prone quads, and calf muscles that they simply don't get a vote in the matter." It would be a mistake to judge Hirsch by his form as he just might pass you.

Hirsch is respectful of his age and the aging process. "The curve plunges," he tells me. He's resigned to not running marathons, and somewhat grateful for his promise to Shay. "It gets hard to keep up the training," he adds. Running has become more social for Hirsch and he looks forward to going to the races and meeting up with friends. It's also a sense of accomplishment. He consistently places in his age group and shoots for an eighty-age-graded percentage. "I love the age-grading! Even when I fall to the back-of-the-pack and revert to a shuffle, I can still compete," says Hirsch.

When asked why he chose running as his life's passion when he could have pursued other sports or ambitions, he doesn't hesitate to respond: "First and foremost, running is a community and the members of this community are some of the most incredible people I have met and am lucky to call friends. We have our own culture, our own leaders, and are dependent on each other for information and advice. . . . It's really one big cocktail party.

"Bill Rodgers is often quoted as saying, 'I've never met a runner that I didn't like, and it's so true. Anyone who can combine a personal passion with a career is ahead of the game. I've never viewed my job at *Runner's World* or New York Road Runners as just a job." He continues his stream of consciousness talking about the friends he has met through the years. "The nature of our sport is communal. I might see someone once a year at a race but when I do, we bond. We're all connected through running and take care of each other. It's the nature of our sport and that's why I love it." He shares a story with me that happened just that morning. He got an email from a man who ran with him at the 1977 New York City Marathon. They met on the course and Hirsch paced him to a PR of 2:40. They stayed in touch for a few years, but Hirsch said they hadn't corresponded in probably twenty-five years. The man reached out to say thanks again for the PR. Hirsch called him and they had a grand old time rehashing the race. "We're still connected through that race after all these years," says Hirsch. "That's what I love about running. I feel so privileged."

We spend more time talking about other aspects that runners share with one another, such as after a race seeing other runners on the subway or the train or even a plane wearing their marathon medal. We get to share our race stories and never tire of telling or hearing them. We look forward to the Olympic marathon event and watch the entire race together.

Hirsch and running have a long history together. Through running he's made lifelong friends, created a career, found his true love, and has traveled the world on behalf of the sport. He leads a simple, fulfilled life and is content. Now that's a goal we should set and achieve.

Sid Howard

DOB: February 6, 1939

Residence: Plainfield, New Jersey

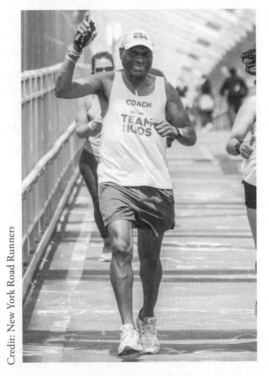

Sid Howard

"Mr. Ambassador of Running."

A high school dropout, married and a father at eighteen, life wasn't easy for Sid Howard. But he persevered and always followed through on what he believed was the right thing to do. He stayed married against all odds and raised six kids. He received his high school equivalency degree and went on to get a college degree at age fifty-nine, with his grandchildren attending his graduation. His stellar track-and-field career includes five world championships, fifty national championships, five world records, and eight World Masters Championships gold medals. Also on his résumé are the American indoor sixty-to-sixty-nine records of 2:19.4 for the 800, 5:23.05 for the mile, and 4:56.36 for 1500 meters. At 79, Howard is running, coaching, and continuing in his unofficial role as ambassador for the sport he loves, and he always has a ready smile and encouraging words for everyone he meets.

Howard is one of ten siblings. His parents migrated from Georgia looking for work and settled in Elizabeth, a factory town in New Jersey just outside Newark. "I don't think my parents ever attended school," says Howard. "We were really poor. My brothers and I slept head to toe in one bed." Due to his parents' long hours at the factory, Howard and his siblings took care of one another. But when his parents were home, they ruled the house with strict discipline. "No one dared cross them or disobey," he recalls. "It wasn't worth the beatings."

He didn't take school seriously, but he was a standout on the track. He was the star runner and thought that his coach would pull rank on his grades. But when he failed math and woodshop his junior year, he was dropped from the team. He could have gone to summer school to make up the classes, but instead he quit school. "Worst decision of my life," says Howard looking back all those years. He joined the Air Force at age seventeen and left his sixteen-year-old girlfriend pregnant when he reported to service. Four years later, at twenty-one, he returned to civilian life and became a husband and father. "I did the right thing. I married her and we went on to have five more babies," says Howard. "We were babies having babies."

For years they worked long hours in the projects, scraping together rent money and teaching their kids the value of an education. They never took a day off, never called in sick. In 1971, Howard got a job driving a truck for a delivery service. It was good pay, the boss trusted him, and things started to look up. Within a few months he went out on his own and has been in business ever since, employing up to twenty-eight people. He continued to be a workaholic, the only way he knew. Having enough money to raise his kids properly was important to him. He and his wife had a successful marriage for thirty-nine years until she died of heart disease in 1997 at the age of fifty-five.

When he was thirty-nine, his son told him there was a mile race in town for "old men like you." Howard hadn't given a thought to running since high school and was tempted to show his kids that "this old dude might still have it." He trained for three weeks and won the race. "My kids were shocked," Howard laughs at the memory. "I didn't even own a pair of running shoes." The race sparked a drive in Howard to return to running. He heard talk about the 1978 New York City Marathon and decided to run it. Since Howard never does anything the easy way, he thought if a marathon was the pinnacle of running, he should shoot for it. He signed up for running classes in Central Park and every Wednesday night ran seventeen miles. Then every morning he would run nine miles on his own. What Howard didn't know at the time was that his running pals were very serious marathoners, who loved to show off their speed at the group runs. "Their idea of a tempo run was to try and drop everyone, leave them in the dust," recalls Howard. Instead of feeling like the newbie he was, Howard embraced it and kept up with the big dogs.

After only three months of training, he was at the starting line of his first marathon, raring to go. His goal was to break three hours. He went out like a flash, weaving around everyone on the Verrazano-Narrows Bridge. He flew for twenty miles and then hit the wall. "Bam! My body revolted and quit," he laughs. By mile 22 he was walking the course in Central Park dazed, disoriented, and starving. He begged for food from the spectators and was given some, which revived him enough to run the last few miles and cross the finish line in 3:02. Instead of calling it quits with the marathon, he was determined to do better, and the next month ran the Jersey Shore Marathon in 3:03. This time, it was the cold that kept him from his sub-three-hour goal. With temperatures below freezing, he didn't know how to dress. Not owning a pair of tights, he wore ladies' panty hose on his legs and a pair of old socks on his hands to keep them from freezing.

He then put in the right training, learned about nutrition and hydration, and finally reached his goal at the 1979 New York City Marathon, running a 2:51. Howard went on to run nine more marathons, with a best time of 2:46:27 in the 1982 New York race, before his love affair with 26.2 miles came to an end. He quit for a number of reasons, mostly because it was just too hard on his body and the training took up too much of his already overscheduled time. "I was juggling the kids, my wife's early stages of heart disease, working all day, and attending college at night," explains Howard. Although he gave up marathons, he kept running. "I start every day with a run, which gives me the energy to get through the day. It continues to be the catalyst for everything I do."

He joined Central Park Track Club in 1978 and started training for shorter distances, where he excelled. When the Fifth Avenue Mile was introduced in 1983 for masters (it began in 1981 for elites only), he entered it and fell in love with the mile. He has since run that race every year, winning his age division for the first time in 1999 at age sixty in 5:12. He has now won his age group at the event a total of ten times, including in 2009, when he ran 5:50 at age seventy.

Turning sixty started an exhilarating year of running for Howard. On his birthday, he set an age-group world record of 2:14.75 for the indoor 800 meters; later that year he set an American masters outdoor record of 2:12.71 at the same distance. Both records lasted for thirteen years. But in the same year, his wife died of heart disease. Her death haunted him because he had tried in vain to get her to exercise and eat healthy food. He's a firm believer that ailments usually associated with aging such as heart disease, stroke, and certain cancers can be prevented with proper diet and exercise. He wasn't always immune to vices, though: he started smoking in high school when he saw his favorite baseball players light up their Lucky Strikes, and later, in the Air Force, "you could always get a break if you said you wanted a cig," he says. He smoked for twelve years and then went cold turkey. He's now a vegetarian and avoids sugar, alcohol, and wheat.

Turning sixty-five began another stellar year for Howard: he won gold medals at 800 and 1500 meters at the 2004 World Masters Indoor Championship in Sindelfingen, Germany. At age sixty-seven, at the World Masters Athletics Indoor Championships in Linz, Austria, he won the 800 meters in 2:28.37 and the 1500 meters in 5:09.42 The following week at the USA Masters Indoor Championships in Boston, he won the mile in 5:37.15 and took second in the 800 in 2:29.85.

In 2005, he married Asteria Claure, a former world-class runner from Bolivia. They make quite a team. Since 2008, they have been coaching for New York Road Runners' charity marathon team, Team for Kids, and have a cadre of first-time marathoners who thank them for their inspiring coaching. They also coach seniors, meeting them at nursing homes and senior centers. He works with a husband and wife at the Midwood Jewish Center in Brooklyn who have been married for seventy years and are ninety-three and ninety-four, respectively. Howard

Photo Album

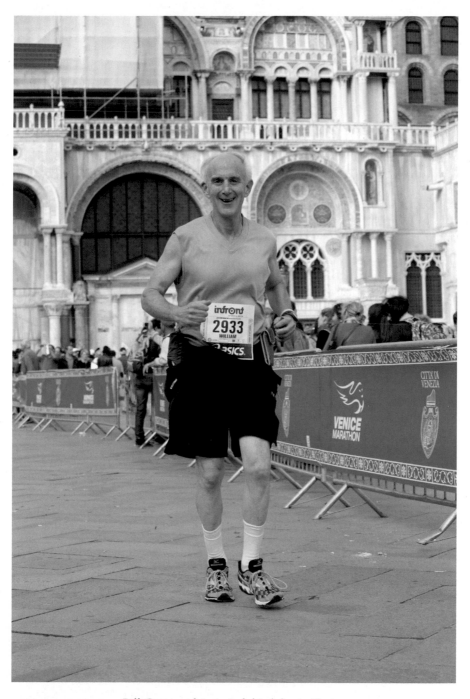

Bill Gross on his sixtieth birthday in Venice

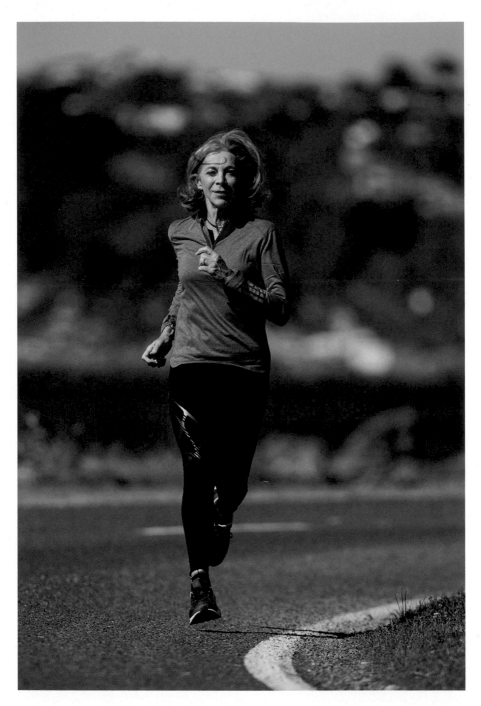

Kathrine Switzer

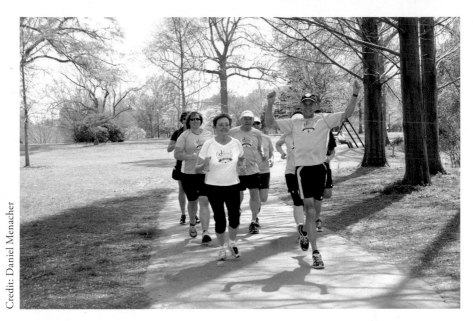

Jeff Galloway

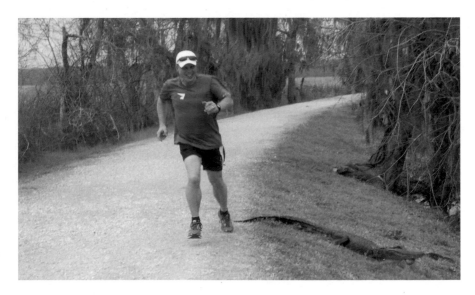

Kevin Follett

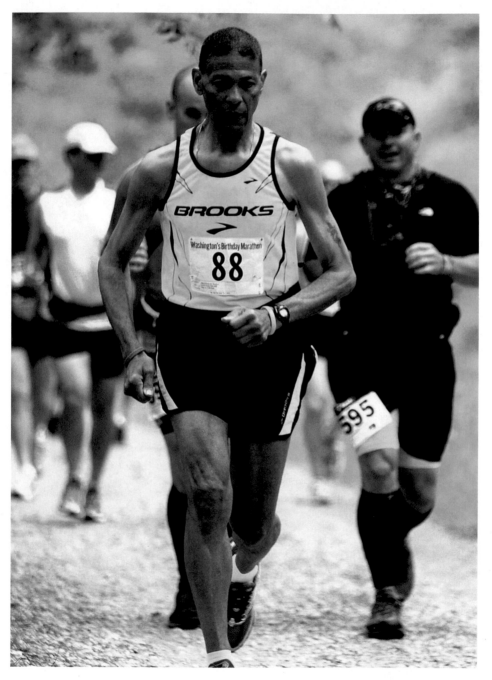

George Banker

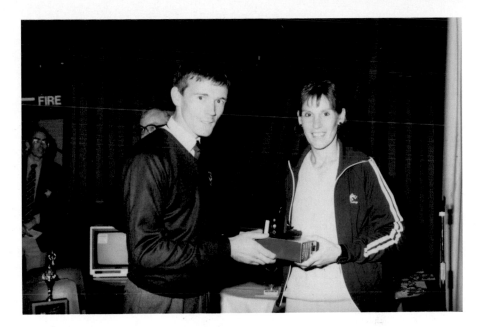

Steve Jones and Karen Bowler, 1985

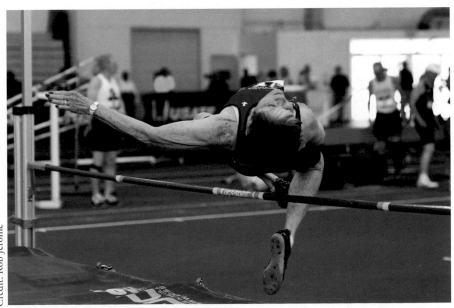

Kathy Bergen

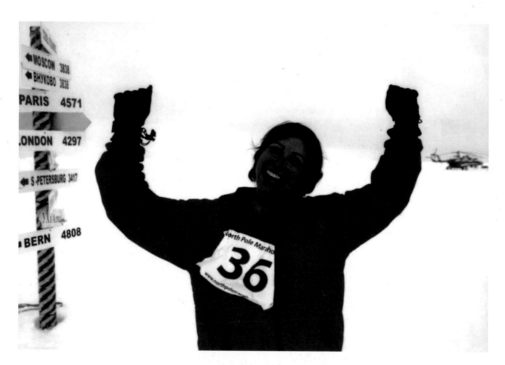

Kimi Puntillo

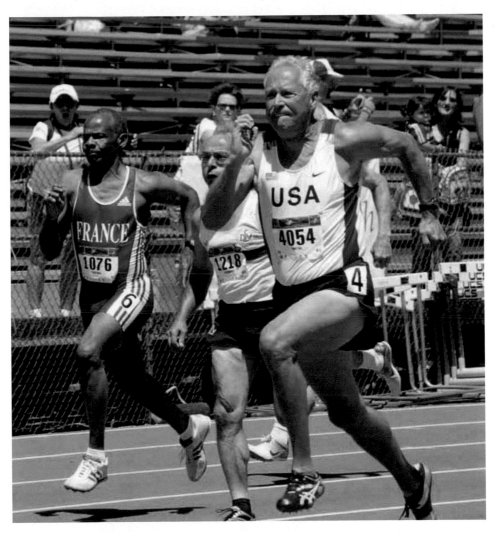

Bob Lida at the World Championships in Sacramento

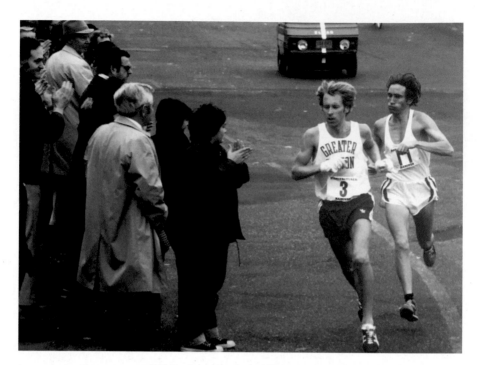

Bill Rodgers at the NYC Marathon

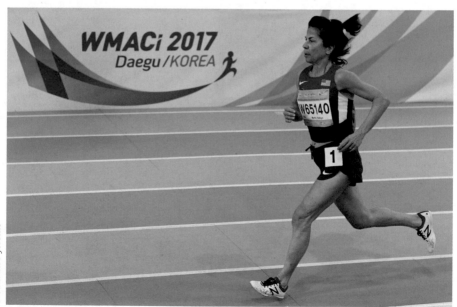

Kathy Martin

gives them chair exercises to build muscle strength and balance and gets them to stretch to help with their flexibility. "It's so rewarding to work with them," says Howard. "I can see the difference these activities make in their lives and they look forward to our sessions."

Howard's running has been put on hold due to an injury in 2014 when he slipped and pulled both hamstrings. But that didn't keep him from running his favorite race, the Bermuda Race series, where he is the only non-Bermudian to receive a bib. He's been running that race for thirty-four years and doesn't plan on missing any of them. His long association with the island's running scene has made Howard in many people's eyes an honorary Bermudian. Running in his distinctive racing cap, he has become instantly recognizable to race spectators who love their honorary member.

In October of 2017, his running club, Central Park Track Club, honored Howard with a dinner at the New York Athletic Club to commemorate his forty years as a member. He was resplendent in a navy-blue-and-white checkered suit, sporting a CPTC baseball cap and a mile-wide smile. Howard is always seen wearing a baseball cap, usually with the New York Yankees logo, his favorite team. The room was packed with hundreds of runners of all ages who came to pay respects to their ambassador of running. He and his CPTC teammates were reminiscing about their US indoor sixty-plus 4×800-meter record of 9:58.0. At the dinner, Nina Kuscsik, the first official female winner of the 1972 Boston Marathon, introduced him. Kuscsik, ever charming and humble about her own legacy, knows a champion when she sees one and was delighted to introduce her old friend. In his speech, Howard thanked all his running buddies and talked about the gift of running and how it has enhanced his life: "Running found me, I didn't find it. It gave me the determination to get through college when I was fifty-nine years old and has rewarded me so many times over. It has taught me to never give up on anything in life. When you suffer during a marathon, and we all suffer, you learn to not listen to the negativity and doubts that start to come around mile 20. You learn to plow through that and come out on top. Running has so many gifts like that and I can't imagine my life without running or my running circle of friends."

Howard and his wife started a tradition a few years ago while visiting her country of Bolivia, one of the poorest in South America. They noticed that the children had to share shoes with their siblings and friends and that they had few or no toys to play with. Moved by their poverty, Howard and Claure started a shoe drive to collect gently-worn running shoes from friends in the tri-state area. At first, they packed the donated shoes in suitcases and took them to Bolivia to distribute, but more shoes kept being donated. Now, they ship the shoes in containers so they can donate more pairs. Each year, they also prepare more than two thousand gift bags filled with healthy snacks—plus dolls for the girls and toy cars and marbles for the boys—and distribute them during Christmas during their annual visit.

As of January of 2018, Howard is still on the injured list, and has tried every physical therapy method available and keeps searching and trying. He keeps up with his coaching by running a twelve-minute pace alongside the runners and calling the drills from the sidelines. He knows how difficult it is to give up winning and setting new records. In 2014, at the World Masters Indoor Championships in Budapest, he and his teammates missed the world record in the 4x800-meter relay by six-tenths of a second. He still runs the Fifth Avenue Mile, although he doesn't always win, and he's okay with that. He's always a crowd-pleaser, win or lose.

Howard's advice for aging runners is to accept that you can't do the speed workouts and quantity of miles that you could before. "It's the quality of the workouts now, not the quantity," he says. "Run every other day and incorporate weight strengthening and balance exercises which become more important as we age." His goal for turning eighty is to get back to competition and start nailing more world and American age-group records. Beyond that, he knows what he'll be doing when he takes his last breath: "My last race will finish at the casket. I'm going to jump in, close the lid, and feel like I lived a full life."

Robert Lida

DOB: November 11, 1936

Residence: Wichita, Kansas

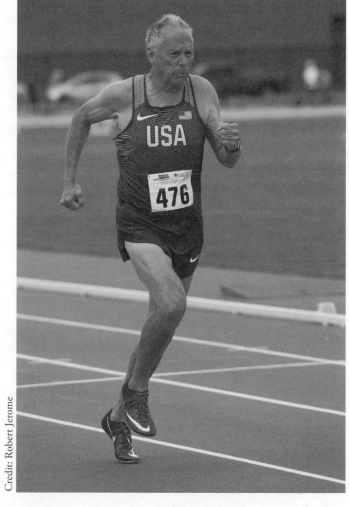

Bob Lida

"I used to be fast. Now I am just fast for my age."

When Ken Stone, athlete, writer, and webmaster of masterstrack.blog suggests I interview someone, I jump on it. He never lets me down and he hit a home run with Bob Lida. When I called Bob at home in Kansas, he had just returned from walking his dog five miles in minus 17-degree weather. That says something about how tough he is but he is also engaging, self-deprecating, and charming. He pushes himself but that's what you have to do to set age group world records. In 2012, seventy-six-year-old Bob Lida, having already accumulated five world records in his age group and been inducted in two Hall of Fames, thought, *I hope I can keep running until I'm eighty. I'm going to keep pushing myself until I can't push any longer. That's what I love to do.*

Now eighty-one, this former University of Kansas sprinter has a total of elven American records and nine world records in the seventy-five-to-eighty age group. He was also selected as the World Masters Athlete best male masters of 2017, adding to his 2012 title of Best Masters of the World award received from the International Association of Athletics Federation in Barcelona, Spain. He's only one of five Americans to receive such an honor and the only American to win it twice.

He's been profiled in the *New York Times,* among other media outlets, not only for his speed but his dedicated work ethic, respect for others, his gracious attitude, and uplifting personality. Lida is laughing at the typical stereotypes of aging—that rocking chair—and is running fast in the opposite direction.

Lida grew up in Kansas City. He credits with his strong belief in being responsible for your actions. "Just remember that what you do will reflect on the entire family," he states. "She [Lida's mother] didn't expect us to win every time but we damn well better have given our all, and she'd know if we didn't." He still hears his mother's voice in his head with that message.

His older brother, ten years his senior, was a great athlete in high school and when Lida came along the coaches were expecting another great Lida athlete. What they got instead was a ninety-eight-pound, short kid who wasn't great at anything. He wanted to play football and had to get a doctor's note to clear him to play because of his size. "What a joke that was," he laughs. His mother bought him football shoes four sizes too large, knowing that sooner or later he'd have a growth spurt. "I can recall stuffing paper towels into the toes of my shoes so I could wear them," he laughs. As a freshman he didn't make the team, but by his junior year he had that growth spurt his mother and tried out again. On the first day of practice during a running drill, he sprinted down the field. When the football coach saw him run, he called the track coach and said, "I think you need to see this kid."

At the University of Kansas, where he was a walk-on for the track team, his teammates included multi All-Americans Wes Santee and Jim Ryan. At first he ran cross country, and "I just couldn't keep up with these guys," he recalls. "But when we ran the 400-meter, I beat them all." The coach decided to switch Lida from cross country to track, where he dominated. From 1957–59 he was a standout sprinter and a Big Eight champion in the indoor 440-yard dash in 1959. In his senior year he suffered a career-ending injury that ended his running for twenty years. "It was an overuse injury that affected my sciatic nerve," explains Lida. He was sidelined for most of his senior year and by the time he got to Nationals, he could barely run at all. "It was so disappointing going from being ranked in the top three or four in the country to being done with my career in one season," says Lida. He lost his motivation to run and compete even when the injury healed. "I just lost the focus," states Lida. He started an advertising company that consumed his time and energy for the next twenty years. By the time he turned forty he had gained weight and was looking for something to get back in shape. That something was masters track.

When he told his father that he was going to start running again, he said, "You know son, you're forty and not as young as you used to be." Lida laughs at this memory. "He believed your heart had so many beats when you got older, then you sat down with the remote and preserved yourself," Lida said. "That was the common view of old age in his generation. You retired and sat in a rocking chair to preserve your heart. You didn't shovel snow, go for long walks or exert yourself in any way."

Lida started running and to this surprise his legs felt fresh. His first meet was in Sweden and he placed eighth in the 400 meter. When he returned home he started training at the local YMCA and fell in with a group of guys who ran marathons. That sounded interesting to him so he trained with the group for the White Rock Marathon, at age forty-three. His competitive spirit came back and he ran three other marathons, eventually breaking the three-hour barrier with a 2:57. He laughs as he recalls his marathon days: "I have a tendency to overdo it. Faster, harder was my go-to method." He ran four marathons until be broke down with hamstring injuries, broken arches, you name it. He was out for four years. When he finally recovered, he went back to road racing, entering 5Ks and 10Ks and stayed on that circuit until age sixty, when he made the switch back to track. "I wanted to see how fast I could make my sixty-year-old body run," says a determined Lida. He started training for the 200-meter and entered his first Senior National Games in Tucson in 1997, taking fifth place. "I was so sore afterwards," recalls Lida. He started training harder and his times dropped.

How is he aging? Lida notes, "To tell you the truth, it's depressing. What bothers me the most is that I still feel sixty but my times are getting slower. My muscles feel like old withered leather. But I'm dealing with it because what else is there? I've reset my goals and am starting to accept my slower times. I'm more selective in how and when I race and the new goal is to leave it all on the track. There's a huge satisfaction in that." He also realizes he has to switch up his training, concentrating more on intensity than volume and trying not to push for that one extra surge that can end with an injury. "Some would say I tend to still push myself," he says with deprecating laughter. "I forget how old I am because I still feel sixty." He tells me a story of how he went too far while hiking in Zion National Park. He signed up for some track events at the October 2017 Huntsman World Senior Games in St. George, Utah, and took a side trip to hike in nearby Zion. He picked a strenuous two-hour climb called Hidden Canyon and then on the way down saw a fork in the trail to Observation Point, an additional six miles. He hadn't taken any water but forged ahead and by the end of the accumulated twelve miles, he suffered for it. "I really hurt my knees and suffered through that for six months," says Lida. "I should have known better but pushed it."

"My sixties were a great decade," says Lida. "I was at the top of my game." In his seventies, he noticed he was slowing down and started concentrating on how his performance matched up against age-graded projections. He also looks at his age-graded percentile as an indicator of his fitness. At seventy-five, while at the World Championships in Finland, he was asked to participate in a study with McGill University in Canada that was comparing seventy-five-year-old sprinters with a peer group of seventy-five-year-olds who did some sports like golf and walking but not training themselves. He was put through a week of testing that included muscle biopsies from the quadriceps and nerve retention in the shin. The results showed that Lida's heart maxed out at a fifty-six-year-old level, meaning sprinters had the heart of a fifty-six-year-olds. "That was good news to me!" exclaimed Lida. Supported by that news, he went on to set two indoor world records in the seventy-five-to-seventy-nine age group, running the 60 meters in 8.49 seconds and the 200 in 27.03. The study also showed that sprinters had more fast-twitch muscle fiber. Lida compared his thigh muscles during the time he was running marathons and said he could put his hands around his thigh. As a sprinter, his leg muscles are much more dense and large. To see Lida run on a YouTube clip means watching a very determined runner who is focused on the finish line. When he finishes, he breaks into a wide smile and turns to congratulate the other runners.

Now in his eighties, he focuses on maintaining balance and flexibility. He notices that some of his friends have installed handrails on their steps and grab bars in the shower, prompted by doctors and advertisements to the senior population. He understands the need for them for some folks but him. "I found myself using the hand rail when I visit them and then thought, heck, I don't need that," he states. "I'd rather use my own balance to get down the stairs." He's always testing himself to see just how far he can push is body. He'll jog up and down the stairs instead of just walking. He stands on one leg when he brushes his teeth. Just for kicks, he hopped up the stairs riser to riser. I tried it and it isn't so easy. "Keep testing yourself and don't give in to the myths of aging," warns Lida. It irritates him when people assume he can't doing something just because of his age. "People defer to me, even my own son warns me at times to slow down," says Lida. "The heck with that."

Lida has a new passion: coaching sprinters and cross country at a local high school. Since 2012 he has coached at Kapaun Mount Carmel. He does the workouts with them and sometimes beats them. His own workouts include Monday and Wednesday sprint drills at 90 to 95 percent effort with Tuesday and Thursday weight strengthening. On Saturdays, he takes the team to run Soap Box Derby Hill, which he compares to a near-death experience but it helps build leg strength and long-speed endurance. On Thursday he runs four sets of bleachers at Wichita State University. Then Sunday at 3:00, he takes his Irish Doodle for a three-mile walk. It seems that Lida gets by on very little sleep. "I take naps," he laughs.

He's most proud of his kids and running a successful advertising agency for thirty years. He also gets a lot of personal reward from the high school kids he coaches who get full scholarships to run at the university level. He also started a new business for removing tattoos. He was inspired by a daughter who wanted her tattoos removed after she became a doctor.

Lida is living a good life. He still trains hard and appreciates every day. He realizes that the next decade will be challenging as friends give up the running scene. "I look ahead at the eighty-five-to-ninety age group and there aren't a lot of guys left," he says on reflection. "Heck, I'll be running against myself!" He also looks at the runners coming up in the ranks and sees a lot of fast ones but is equally reflective of the fact that his records will be broken. "All records are temporary," he states matter-of-factly.

What has become more important to Lida as he ages is the social aspect and camaraderie of attending masters championships and senior games. In a profile of Lida on the December 2017 National Senior Games Associate website, Lida provides the main reason he shows up at senior games, and it isn't what you might think: "I want to win, and I prepare hard to win. My goal today is to beat the age curve. But that's not why I show up," he explains. "There's a common bond that you have when you are in masters track. I have made long friendships in this country, and also in places like Germany, England, and Australia. We keep in touch and it's great to see them at world championships every year."

His goal moving forward is simple: "Keep doing what I do. That will keep me happy for the rest of my life."

Betty Lindberg

DOB: September 7, 1924

Residence: Atlanta, Georgia

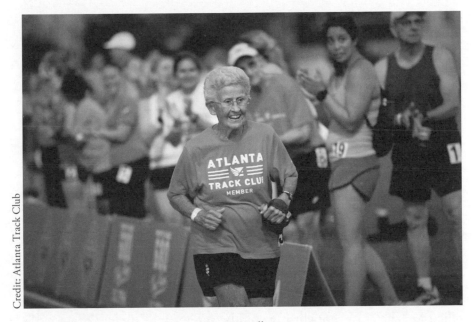

Betty Lindberg

I'm Still Here!

In 2016, Betty Lindberg set a world record and USATF record in the 800 meters for women ninety-to-ninety-four with a time of 6:57.56. In May of 2017, at age ninety-two, she set a USATF record for the women's ninety-plus division in the 400 meters in 3:05.01, shattering the twenty-one-year-old record of 3:45.62. Two months later, she won her age group at the Peachtree Road Race in a time of 2:22.46. This Georgia senior is charming, spirited, and full of vim and vigor. A beloved member of the Atlanta Track Club, Lindberg is up for anything except the pole vault. She does not let her age define her. "Age is just a number," says Lindberg. "Act how you feel."

When I call Betty at her Atlanta home, she has just come in from hanging Christmas decorations on the house. "The neighbors get real scared when they see me on the ladder," she laughs. She tells me she wears hearing aids and asks me to speak a little louder than normal. "When I meet people and can't hear them, I just smile and nod," she explains. That would be a shame, as she has a lot to say and it's all very interesting.

Lindberg was born in Minnesota and graduated from high school in 1942. She wanted to go to college and become a teacher but the War was on and she wanted to do her part to help out. "We were already saving soup cans and newspapers like everyone did but I wanted to do more," said Betty. She joined the National Youth Association, a government sponsored program that taught civilians occupational training to help the war effort, and she learned Morse code. After the war, those skills landed her a job with Northwest Airlines where she met her future husband, Lindy, during a company hayride. They moved to Atlanta in 1958, and she fell into the role of a happy homemaker and mother. She was never active or played sports. "Girls didn't partake in any activity that would make them sweat!" she recalls. "I hopscotched." While her kids were in school, she worked part-time as an administrative assistant at a department store, at a time when most women did not work outside of the house. When asked if she needed the job as secondary income, she relied no, she "just thought it would be interesting." Being interested is a trait that Betty carried throughout her life and defined her. In high school, she joined the photography club because she thought it would be interesting and loved learning to work a Brownie camera. "I like to try things," she tells me. "Why lead a dull life? There's so many things to try and see if you like it. Just give it a try. So what if you fall on your face? At least you tried."

That spunk and curiosity is what led her to running. She can recall the day that she got interested in running. She was sixty-three at the time and drove her daughter and son-in-law to the Peachtree Road Race, a

10K held on July 4. "I never even heard of this race but they wanted to do it, so I agreed to drive them to the start. I really wanted to go back to bed but promised to see them at the finish," she says. She was inspired by the wheelchair athletes who finished first, then was awed by the pros who sped by. Then she watched the mob of mid-packers go by and thought, "I can do this." Determined, when she got home she decided to walk two blocks, more activity than she'd done in a long time. "I got to the end of the two blocks and didn't think I'd make it home," she laughs.

Betty is not one to quit and did that walk every day until she could do it without stopping. She joined the Atlanta Track Club (ATC), becoming the oldest member, and was welcomed by everyone. Today she is a cherished and protected participant. When reporters call looking for Lindberg, they are met with questions and vetted to make sure they are worthy enough to speak with her.

With the backing and support of ATC, the following year she entered and completed the Peachtree Road Race, her first race, at age sixty-four. In July 2017, she finished her twenty-seventh Peachtree Road Race, making her the oldest participant to finish. There were five people over ninety, Lindberg and four males, but Lindberg edged out the ninety-two-year-old man by a week. "I beat two of the ninety-one-year-old kids. Can you imagine!" she says with glee.

Her fame has garnered her celebrity status. At races she is asked to pose for selfies, which she says slows her down a bit but she accommodates. Her 2016 time was 1:51:43, faster than her 2:22:46 (more selfies) in 2017. She's now sponsored by Mizuno, the sports equipment, shoe, and gear provider.

When she turned seventy-one she decided to become a race walker and joined the Walking Club of Georgia. She completed a few half-marathons using their program. In 2016, at the ATC All-Comers, an event for any ability and any age, Lindberg ran the 800-meter. She had no idea there was a record for the event. "I just wanted to finish two laps around the track before they put out the lights," she recalls. "Coming down the last 100 meters I heard everyone cheering for me. 'Come on, Betty! You can do it!' I thought they were just pleased I finished without killing myself."

The next morning, she received a call from the director of the ATC with the news that she had set a world record for her age group by two seconds. "I was completely surprised," says Lindberg. "I had no idea."

Everyone in her family was also shocked and pleased. Her nephew said, "Old people are always breaking things but not world records!" In May of 2017, she decided to go for the 400-meter record at the All Comers meet. This time was different. She knew what time she needed to beat. "I couldn't hide," she says. "I felt a lot of stress."

She stood alone in lane four and recalls the moment: "When I walked up to the start, I thought, I don't want to disappoint anyone. I'm going to give it my best." And she did, beating the existing record by over forty seconds. Her cheering section went wild as she approached the finish line but she was concentrating so hard she barely heard them.

At ninety-three, Lindberg feels pretty good. She reflects on aging: "Everyone is going to die at some point, I'm just not ready. The big truck hasn't mowed me down yet." She credits good genes for aging successfully. She's had no serious injuries to speak of but did have a hip replacement in 2014 at eighty-nine. "I was bone on bone and on a walker," she recalls. "Best decision I ever made and afterward thought why did I wait so long?" Earlier that year, not wanting to end her Peachtree Road Race streak, she recieved a cortisone shot and walked the race that year.

Reaching out to her son Craig, he added these comments about his mom: "Mom was raised during the Depression Era and her parents, Henna and Clyde Reynolds, were not well off and worked very hard. Everyone did chores. They had a wringer washer to clean their clothes and a wood-burning stove. It was a big deal when they got a Ford Model-A. Her parents ran a diner (Mom collected the eggs from the henhouse out back) and then a boarding house, and then Clyde worked at a lumber yard before finally getting a job with the draft board; he actually inducted his son Bob, Mom's brother, into the army at the start of World War II, where he saw combat with the 10th Mountain Division. Her parents built the only house they ever owned, using wood and nails from a barn they disassembled stick by stick as you couldn't get building materials during the War. Because it was miles away and gasoline was rationed, they lived in a tent by a pond where they slept, cooked, and bathed while they built the house, hauling the materials to the home site. Indeed her upbringing, but also the era when she grew up, shaped her. The breadth of change she's seen in her years is pretty hard to comprehend." Craig adds her sense of humor to the list of items that he loves about his mom that contributes to keeping her youthful.

Betty admits to some memory loss and makes sure to write things down. She follows a healthy diet. But the biggest advice she gives is to have a healthy attitude and to keep moving. She laughs and is upbeat during our conversation and in every photo I see of her, she is sporting a huge engaging smile. "I feel well," she exclaims throughout our talk. "I get out and move every day to keep the blood flowing and I feel exhilarated." In 2006, her husband of fifty-seven years passed away and she has lived alone since but she is surrounded by family nearby. Although she doesn't need assistance when shopping or going out in general, she understands that people who don't know her see her as "a little gray-haired old lady who needs help" and open doors for her and help her in and out of her car. She's polite to them but chuckles inwardly that she's probably in better shape then they are. She admits to losing some motivation last year when her left knee starting aching. She used the pain as an excuse not to run and got lazy. "The twinge scared me but it wasn't that bad. Basically, I just got lazy and that bothered me," she says. "I was ashamed of myself and had to kick my own butt to get motivated again. I never want to be a quitter."

On January 1, 2018, she signed up for the ATC's one-mile Resolution Run but when she woke up the temperature was 17 degrees, unseasonably cold for Atlanta. She dressed anyway and headed to the event, but when she stepped out of her car, the cold wind hit her face and falling tears froze on her cheeks. She states, "I decided to go back home!" She finally completed her resolution race in April at the Atlanta Track Club's annual Northside Hospital Atlanta Women's 5K. "It's just a real fun race and I love that it is all women out there," she says. She's been working with a personal trainer three times a week focusing on strength training and balance. She can hold a plank for seventy-five seconds and does eighty-pound dead lifts as part of her routine along with sit-ups, push-ups, and anything else to get her stronger. "Balance is tricky for old people," states Lindberg. "I really have to look where I put my feet."

Her motto is "Make No Excuses." "I don't want to be a postscript where people say, 'What happened to Betty?' Heck, I'm still here!"

James Manno

DOB: November 10, 1920

Residence: Pompton Plains, New Jersey

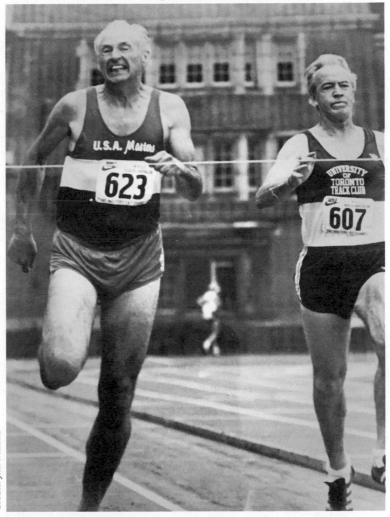

Credit: Jim Manno

The 1981 North American championships in Philadelphia. Here Jim (left) sets a new 200m meet record M60 in twenty-seven seconds.

"What a journey!"

Jim Manno knows what it's like to hear the sound of forty-eight thousand spectators cheering him on at the 2001 Penn Relays. Then eighty, he won his age group in the 100-meter. "I can close my eyes and still picture that day," says Manno, ninety-seven at the time of our interview. "The sound of the crowds will never leave my memory." Manno had a nice stretch of competing for over seventy years before hanging up his spikes for good at age ninety-one. He still goes to the track twice a week to stay in shape and keep his college-age weight. He still drives a 1999 Cadillac Eldorado two-door silver coupe and has no plans to relinquish his license soon although he doesn't drive at night anymore. Why should he? He's as sharp as a tack.

James Manno was raised in Union City, New Jersey, during the Depression. His father owned a handbag factory and worked six and a half days a week to keep a roof over their heads and food on the table. His mother worked alongside his father at the factory. Recalls Manno, "They did everything they could to save a dime." Manno had jobs as well, cleaning the house after school, then sweeping the floors of the factory when that was done and going home to prepare dinner for his sister and parents. "There was no time for games or playing with friends," says Manno. "I wanted to run track in high school but didn't have the time."

He does recall his very first race, in grammar school. It was an all-day track-and-field event for all the public schools in the area. Schools were identified by a colored banner that each child wore across their T-shirt. Manno was running the 50-yard dash and when he went to the start line, his classmates cheered for him. But when he finished second to last, he got booed by the same kids. "I learned early in life how fickle spectators can be!"

Manno finally got his chance to run track in college at New York University. As a sophomore walk-on he started to score points for his team and was recognized as a talented half-miler. His teammates included Leslie MacMitchell, a gifted runner who received the AAU James E. Sullivan Award, the top US award for amateur athletes, in 1941. MacMitchell also gained a share of the world record for an indoor mile run. "With teammates like that, I always took second or third place but what an honor to be on the same team," states Manno.

By his senior year he was attending national meets in Syracuse and Boston running the two-mile relay. That same year he won a race in

Madison Square Garden, a 1,000-yard handicap. His picture was in the *New York Times* and he still has that paper and medal. "That was my first big win and I can still recall the eighteen-thousand spectators cheering for me," says Manno. "I never thought I could top that experience in my life." But he did. At age eighty he won the 100-yard dash at the 2001 Penn Relays. "I never experienced such a thrill," states Manno. "I was trying to win that gold watch since 1941!" The headlines in his local paper the next day read, "60 years later Manno gets his gold watch."

During his senior year of college, Pearl Harbor was attacked. After completing college, Manno enlisted in the Coast Guard, spending the next four years aboard ship in the Pacific. His first ship escorted convoys in the Atlantic. After Germany surrendered, he was transferred to the Pacific to another ship that was practicing for the invasion of Japan when the war ended. He returned home in 1946, got married in 1948, got a job, and started to earn a living. He began jogging at a local high school track, doing 100s and 200s. In 1975 at age fifty-six, now living in Oradell, New Jersey, with two sons and a daughter, he read an article about a track meet in Piscataway, New Jersey. Interested to see what the track scene was like all these years later, he took his fifteen-year-old son to the meet. Manno saw men his age participating and said to his son, "I think I can beat them." To which his son replied rather snarkily, "Yeah, sure you can dad." That's all Manno needed to hear. He was up to the challenge thrown down. He found a track meet the following weekend at Randall's Island in Manhattan, dug out his old college spikes, and went to the meet, returning home with two first place trophies in the 220 and 440 meters.

His adrenaline spiking, Manno started working out like crazy, attending every track meet he could find. He trained three days a week and on weekends at a local high school track just down the street from his house. That year, his comeback year after thirty-three years, he won two state championships. He self-coached, studying what others did. He found fartleks to be his key workout and entered 5Ks. "I never won but the race atmosphere and speed really helped my track. The 100, 200, and 400 meters were my staple," recalls Manno. He traveled the eastern seaboard for meets, driving to Syracuse, Boston, Raleigh, North Carolina, and Philadelphia. "I lived in the car," laughs Manno.

In 1976, he read an article about an upcoming track meet in New York for masters runners. Excited to participate, he made a few phone calls and was led to Fred d'Elia in Ridgewood, New Jersey, for more information. That phone call changed Manno's life. D'Elia was a masters track runner and lived in the next town from Manno. D'Elia's wife, Toshiko (Toshi), was a world-class distance runner, the first female in the world to run a sub-three-hour marathon at age fifty in the world masters championships. At forty-nine, she completed the Boston Marathon in 2 hours, 58 minutes, and 11 seconds. Over the years she broke many age-group records up until her death at age eighty-four. Mary Wittenberg, then president of New York Road Runners, called her "the queen of the roads." From 1976 to 2011 Fred, Toshi, and Manno bonded over their passion for running and traveled together every weekend to meets and races. Together they founded North Jersey Masters, a running club in northern New Jersey, and put on a Memorial Day run that is still one of the largest races in New Jersey. "We were like family," says Manno. "I miss them."

In his fifties and sixties, Manno was on a roll, setting world and national records. At age eighty, he set a world record in the 200 meters indoors in 32.85 seconds. Ironically, d'Elia held that record for ten years before Manno broke it. In all, Manno won twenty-seven national championships and four gold medals as part of a sprint medley relay.

I ask Manno why track? "Behind every track man is a frustrated basketball, football, or baseball player," laughs Manno. "If you can't make those teams, you go out for track where everyone is accepted." On a more serious note, he states that he had a passion for track and knew he was good at it. With his Depression-era work ethic, training hard came easy. "I enjoyed the hard work," Manno says. "And the sprint distances were a lot easier than training for a 5K." When he traveled for work, he brought his spikes and when his co-workers hit the bar, he hit a local track. He credits Helen, his "very patient wife," as the biggest reason he was able to do what he did. "She was agreeable to my weekend travels and gave me the support I needed," says Manno. His running community of Fred, Toshi, and others became his second family. Manno has wonderful memories of his career on the track. He tells me the story of setting the world indoor record for the M80 200-meter at Boston in 2001. Before he went to the event he looked up the American record and thought he had a chance of breaking it. As he approached the finish line tape, the announcer was enthusiastically screaming that Manno would set an American record. When he finished and broke the record, spectators in the stands came down to the track to congratulate him. "One young woman was crying, she was so happy for me," recalls Manno. It wasn't till he arrived home the next day that he found out he also set a world record.

Manno quit competing at age ninety-one. His last meet was in 2011. "I had trouble even jogging the 400," he recalls. "Plus most of my competitors are dead." He looks around his study at all his photos framed on the wall of his track days with his friends and points out, "this one is dead, and that one is dead. Heck, I'm the last guy standing." Just the year before at age ninety, he ran four races, winning gold in the 200 meters at the World Championships in Sacramento. After that he noticed his times slowing. At his last meet in Ohio, he placed second and was frustrated with his performance. "I was getting too old for all the travel and the toll it takes to attend the meets," states Manno. "I think I was just tired after all the years."

Manno didn't want to be a second place competitor. For him, it was do your best and win or don't bother showing up. He had a great career, representing the United States at world competitions five times and accumulating a lifetime achievement of 463 gold medals, 134 silver, and forty bronze. Plus a gold watch from the Penn Relays. And tons of memories. He tells a story of competing in Canada and driving back after his meet and facing difficulty at the border crossing. At customs, he was asked why he was in Canada and he responded that he was running in a track meet. "The border agent looked at my gray hair and kind of gave me a look that implied I was lying, but after a while just waved me on," laughs Manno at the memory.

In 2013, Manno and his wife moved from their home in Oradell, New Jersey, to a retirement community in Pompton Plains. Moving out of their house after fifty-three years was a bit traumatic as he took on the task of sorting through hundreds of medals and trophies, photographs, old but beloved spikes, and memories. What to keep and what to throw out became a daily exercise. He also left his favorite track at River Dell High School, right down the street from his house and where he was a favorite fixture and inspiration to the students. A scholarship was established by North Jersey Masters at River Dell in Manno's name for seniors on the track and cross country teams.

His decision to move to a retirement community was well thought out and a good one for Manno and his wife. Cedar Crest is far from "an old peoples' home" as we used to call facilities for seniors. According to Manno, "Cedar Crest is like a college campus. We have thirteen apartment houses, with about eighteen hundred retirees, four restaurants, three libraries, three beauty salons, two gyms, an indoor swimming pool, and over a hundred different clubs and activities to join." That keeps Manno busy, along with his track workouts.

"I've been very successful in my career so I have no regrets about quitting," he explains. "Heck, who takes up track at age fifty-five and has the time of his life not only winning but meeting lifelong friends? I don't want to put in the work to stay on top anymore," he states. "I knew it was over for me when it became work and not fun." He is most proud of representing the US in five world championships and winning two gold medals and five silvers in world championship meets. Now track is a hobby, not a career. He goes to the gym and works out on the treadmill on the days he doesn't go to the track. Occasionally he'll get comments from folks who mean well when they say something like, "Good for you! Keep it up!" Manno doesn't like that. "I know what they are really thinking is look at that old man trying to stay in shape," he says with sarcasm. He's learning to take it in stride and resists telling the young whippersnappers that he was once a top competitor who represented the United States in world competitions.

Aging isn't easy, especially when inside you still feel like that warrior on the track. One of the best lessons we can learn from aging is to accept who we are at every age. Manno embraces his age but doesn't want to be perceived as an old geezer. And thanks to seniors like Manno and others that follow, they are changing people's attitudes about aging. Also important is that Manno feels he is still in control. He takes care of his wife, cooks meals, and puts in a full day. At ninety-seven, he could actually take a little more time to relax and rest but that's not in his DNA. He could probably still kick the butt of guys half his age in a 100 meter, but he is now happy to run for fun. He deserves that.

Gerald Miller

DOB: March 8, 1937

Residence: Calgary, Alberta, Canada

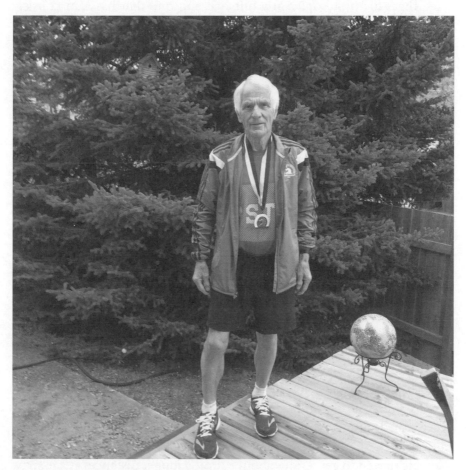

Jerry Miller

"A bundle of energy at eighty."

Gerry Miller and I connect from his home in Calgary via a FaceTime call. It's early in the morning and he has already gone for his daily run. He's wearing his Boston Marathon shirt from 2017 and moves around a lot on our call, giving me a tour of his house and his medal wall. For most of the call he paces back and forth in the living room, occasionally sitting on the couch for a few minutes before he's up again. He believes in the power of moving. "Get up every day and get moving," he says. "If you're moving, you work better mentally, spiritually, and your body definitely works better."

That's his philosophy in a nutshell and one that has him consistently winning or placing in his eighty-to-eighty-four age group. At the 2017 Boston Marathon, he came in second with a time of 4:32:54. If he knew there was a competitor somewhere ahead of him, he would have tried harder, but then again, he says with his usual positivity, "You never know what the day is going to bring. I'm just glad I'm still here."

Miller grew up on a farm near Galahad in east-central Alberta, Canada, with a twin brother. By age four they both were doing farm chores like tilling the land, hauling rocks, and milking cows. It was a very rural area, and they were poor. He attended a one-room schoolhouse for elementary school, riding a horse to get there before his family moved closer to town. During his summers he worked on a drilling rig in Edmonton, which built his strength. After high school, he attended the University of Alberta, obtaining a degree in engineering. At the university he played hockey to stay active.

After graduating, he got a job teaching at the University of Calgary as an education professor. He was married and had four kids. He coached his kids' soccer teams, hockey teams, jogged around the university campus, and basically kept moving to stay in shape. "I've been moving all my life, I never stop," says Miller. Life was good for Miller. He was happy, loved his job, his kids, and his wife. When his kids were old enough to run six miles, he ran a local Mother's Day 10K with them just about every year. That was the extent of his running, besides his jogging around campus.

He started to get serious about running longer distances at age sixty, when his son convinced him to join him on a nineteen-mile run with a local running club that was training for the Vancouver Marathon. After the nineteen-miler, Miller felt fresh enough to keep up the training and ran the 2003 Vancouver Marathon, his first, and qualified for Boston with a 3:54. "I was over-the-top excited," recalls Miller. He also recalls how sore he was after the 26.2 miles, walking backward down the steps to the food tent to get his cookies and banana. "I was such a newbie I didn't even wear a watch," laughs Miller. I didn't know anything about running marathons but now I wanted to know everything." He was exhilarated at finishing his first marathon. "I did the impossible!" he exclaims.

He started running two or three marathons a year, some with his sons. On his fireplace mantle is a photo of him and one of his sons at the finish line of the Rock 'n' Roll Las Vegas Half Marathon they ran together. Miller is a committed family man and now grandfather. His favorite marathons are Boston and New York City. His most memorable is the 2013 Boston Marathon. On April 15, 2013, Miller could not have imagined his race would end with a bomb going off at the finish line when he was just yards from the finish. He was running next to his friend Bill Ifrigg, who went down from the blast. He recalls that day: "We had turned onto Boylston Street. I was right behind Bill when the bomb went off, knocking him down. We all stopped in our tracks, not quite realizing what had happened. A big Irish cop came over and led us from the course. I had no money or clothes and couldn't get to my bags. I was so cold and now crying and shaken from what I was seeing. A woman came over and draped a blanket around me, another gave me water and let me borrow her cell phone. Everyone was so generous and caring to the runners. It still brings tears to my eyes when I think of it. Runners are part of a wonderful community, and we all came together that day along with the generous spectators." He went back and ran in 2014, finishing in 4:05 at age seventy-seven, buoyed by the support and love he received from the spectators.

Miller has not only logged thousands of miles at races, but he has also logged thousands of hours as a volunteer at race events. In 2015, he received the North American Volunteer of the Year Award presented by Running Room Canada. He also received the Top 7 over 70 Award in 2017 for making a difference within the province of Alberta. Miller shows me the photos taken at the gala and he is beaming, looking elegant in a tuxedo. "Running is a blessing I want to share, so I love to volunteer and help out as much as I can," he says. "It's my way of giving back for everything running has given me."

Now a retired professor, Miller dedicates most of his days to training and staying fit for his marathons. Starting out strong in his sixties, he noticed a slight slowing of his times in his seventies. He changed his routine a bit, adding more cross-training like spin classes and doing less rigorous speed workouts. "I try to maintain a decent pace so I have enough piss and vinegar at the end to sprint across the finish," he adds. His finish-line sprints have earned him first age at the 2017 Berlin Marathon and two months later at the New York City Marathon finishing in 4:34 at age eighty.

He enjoys his spin classes, which he does three times a week. "I'm the old man with the young moms," he laughs. He also loves to hike the trails near his home and thinks nothing of a four-hour trek. He chops and carries his own firewood. "I do anything I can to create resistance to the muscles and keep moving," says Miller. He also maintains a healthy diet, starting his day with chia seeds, hemp hearts, and full-fat yogurt. His go-to snack is coconut oil mixed with peanut butter, spread on a rye crisp. "It's delicious!" he adds. "What we put in our gut makes a big difference in our health." He credits his upbringing on the farm with his ability to run strong and be in a winning position. "At an early age on the farm, my twin brother and I were picking roots, rocks, cleaning the barn, and excelling within a small community school. I developed a rather Type-A personality," he explains. "Running is also my personal space, an enjoyable activity that helps me relax."

He's never been injured and credits that to stretching and going out slowly. "It's time on your feet, not speed, that will keep you out there longer," he explains. His advice to first-time marathoners as well as aging marathoners is to just relax, feel blessed to be running at all, and have a great time. At his age, running has also become a social outlet where he meets old friends and catches up with running buddies he sees maybe once a year at races. "I enjoy the camaraderie of seeing friends at events," says Miller. "We joke about still being here, and we have a few laughs. It's worth every minute I spend with them."

He gives lectures on living a healthy lifestyle and the "power within" to running groups. He paces first-time runners at races and thoroughly enjoys the experience. "I encourage people by talking to them and laughing a lot," he explains. "I think they get a kick out of being paced by an eighty-year-old." He is what they call a pace bunny at his club because the pace leaders wear a white cap with pink bunny ears. "Okay, go figure. I wear my ears with pride," he laughs. He's been a pace leader for ten years and loves the experience. He is a big believer in building confidence in new runners.

Miller is having a lot of fun with his running. He was part of a group that set a Guinness World record for the most runners linked at the 2017 Calgary Marathon. Using four feet of surgical tubing, 112 runners stayed together for the 26.2 miles. "If one of us went down, we all went down," laughs Miller. The group had three planned bathrooms breaks and finished in 6:24. His next goal is to be the first eighty-year-old to complete all six of the Abbott World Marathon Majors, each one in under five hours. He has London and Tokyo left to do and is looking for sponsors to help him with the expenses.

Miller is humbled by his late-in-life accomplishments. It's almost like he is experiencing a second coming of his life and is enjoying every minute of it. His exuberance is contagious. At his marathons he wears a shirt with the inscription "Canada 80+" on the back. He gets touches on his shoulders from well-wishers throughout his races, which he thinks makes him run faster. "It is a blessing to do what I do," Miller says. "Every day is a gift."

Charles Milliman

DOB: November 14, 1932

Residence: Sequim, Washington

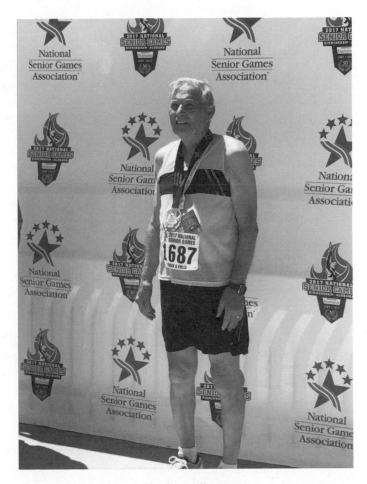

Charles Milliman

"Eighty-five miles on his eighty-fifth birthday."

Chuck Milliman is not your average octogenarian. In fact, he's probably not your average anything. On his seventy-eighth birthday, he ran seventy-eight miles. That was so much fun he ran eighty miles on his eightieth birthday and in 2018 ran eighty miles on his eighty-fifth birthday. When he's not running, he is practicing the pole vault in a backyard pit that he built with his son. This retired pastor knows how to live a fulfilled life. With Shirley, his wife of sixty-seven years, by his side, there doesn't seem to be much that Milliman can't do once he sets his mind to it.

When I call Milliman for the interview, his voice is so steady and youthful that I think I have the wrong number. But he jumps on the call and says, "Are you the person writing a book about crazy people?" His wife is in the background chiming in, "You may be sorry you called!" This is my introduction to Chuck and Shirley.

Milliman grew up in Hooper, Washington, during the Depression, where his family managed a sheep ranch. The town had a general store and a one-room schoolhouse. That's it. The town still exists today and has a population of twenty-one. One of six siblings, he and two older siblings attended the one-room schoolhouse; the three Milliman kids, two other children, and the school teacher's daughter were the only kids in the classroom from first through eighth grade. Their home had no electricity or running water. "Going to the outhouse in zero degrees was tough," laughs Milliman of his childhood. To earn extra money, he and his brother picked wool off dead sheep to sell in town. For fun, they tore pages from the Sears Roebuck Catalogue and made paper airplanes. "We were very isolated," says Milliman. "But we had a roof over our heads and food on the table so we were happy. We didn't know any better." When Pearl Harbor was attacked, their neighbors drove over in their car and they all piled in so they could listen to the news. To this day, that Depression-era mentality still sticks. Milliman never throws anything out.

Then the family moved south of Spokane in the spring of 1944. In the spring, he and his two older siblings took a train down to Benton City to cut asparagus in the fields for local farmers (he was all of twelve years old). In 1946 when he was in the eighth grade, his family moved to Benton City, Washington. Graduating from Benton City High School in 1951, he married his high school sweetheart, Shirley.

He "stumbled through life" doing numerous odd jobs: construction worker, butcher, laying railroad ties, and numerous other odd jobs. He was also taking college correspondence courses in electronics, which ultimately led to a job with Boeing in Seattle where he worked for five years. During this time, he did a lot of thinking about God. *Is this all there is to life, punching in my hours at work?* he would ask himself. The question lingered in his head that spring through August as he felt pulled toward a life in the ministry. In 1963, he answered the calling and enrolled in Warner Pacific College, a Christian liberal arts school in Portland. "Shirley and I plus our three children all agreed to the plan," states Milliman. Shirley worked fulltime while he studied and worked part-time. He was ordained in 1970.

Throughout the years Milliman stayed active hiking along Mount Hood in Oregon with Shirley and the kids. One of Milliman's professors, who was in his late sixties, was an avid hiker who knew all the trails around Mount Hood and eventually, Milliman, his kids, and the professor all climbed Mount Hood. While out hiking one day the professor mentioned that he ran the Trails End Marathon earlier that spring of 1972. Milliman's reaction was, "If this old man can run marathons, I can." He talked to his sons, already runners on their high school track and cross-country teams, about training for a marathon and in the fall of 1972, he began his training.

Milliman and his sons all signed up for the Trails End Marathon in Seaside, Oregon and started training. In February 1973, he toed the line of his first marathon at age forty. Despite all the training, by mile 20 he was crying like a baby, cursing himself for signing up. "I felt like a big dummy, totally out of my element," he recalls. "I swore I would never do this again." He finished in 3:59. The following morning, somewhat recovered, he became elated with his accomplishment and read a proverb from the Bible: "Weeping happens at night, Joy cometh in the morning." He now has a twenty-five-year streak at that marathon.

After taking a three-week recovery, he was back running 10Ks. The next year, he ran three marathons and continued doing that into his seventies. The entire family got into running marathons and did many together throughout the years. If there was a family division, they always took first place.

Meanwhile, his son Philip who pole vaulted in high school picked it up again at age fifty. He entered the senior state games in pole vault and persuaded his dad to come along. Why not?! Father and son built a pole vault pit in their backyard so they could practice. At age seventy-two, at the 2004 National Senior Games, Milliman vaulted over six feet, taking first place. He continued to practice and in 2017 at age eighty-five he vaulted over five feet, ten inches to win a gold medal. He also competed in the high jump, taking first place. He plans to compete next year when "There are fewer athletes in my age division so I can usually come in at the top five," laughs Milliman. "So I always get a medal!" From the background, I can hear Shirley yelling at him not to be so vain.

Milliman is an unbeatable athletic machine, but he's had his down-turns. In 2001, at age sixty-nine, he underwent heart bypass surgery to correct two arteries that were 95 percent blocked. He didn't run another marathon until 2007. "The surgery wasn't related to running so I don't count it as an injury," jokes Milliman. He hasn't been to a doctor in years, part of his Depression-era mentality. "Who has the time or money to go a doctor?" He credits his injury-free running with not obsessing about time or distance. "I just like to have fun with my running," he explains. "I really believe that by surrounding myself with family and friends who run with me, that I don't get any injuries. We are having too much fun." He doesn't stretch or cross-train and don't even ask about massages or gym memberships. He hikes, rides a bike, and eats whatever Shirley makes him. "My wife is good at cooking healthy meals," he says proudly.

To celebrate his seventy-eighth birthday, he ran three marathons in three days to raise funds for the Boys & Girls Club of Sequim, Washington. He jokes, "I decided that after paying out all those race fees it was time someone paid me to run!" He marked a 26.2-mile course through his neighborhood and ran from 9:00 a.m. to 4:00 p.m. every day, by himself, and raised $3,000. "It wasn't a big deal," he says with deprecating humor. "I felt fine." For his eightieth birthday he decided to run eighty miles and again, raise funds for the Boys & Girls Club. He started that adventure at midnight on November 14 in 40-degree weather and ran until 11:50 p.m. on November 15, finishing in twenty-three hours and fifty minutes. He was accompanied by his son-in-law, Dick, for the first thirty miles and then his grandson, Jason, covered the remaining fifty miles with him. He also had support from another son, Bruce, and another grandson, Doug. Following in a motor home was his support crew: his daughter, Kim, and son, Phillip. Shirley waited nervously at home.

At sixty miles he stopped for a latte and had some arthritis cream rubbed on his knee. In the middle of the night, his grandson fed him bagel bites. "I was slow," recalls Milliman. "I was averaging 2.5 miles per hour for the last twenty miles. But my support crew were unbelievable and got me through it." The crew backed off the final two-tenths of a mile so he could finish solo. The executive director of the Boys & Girls Club called him an inspiration for all ages.

Five years later at eighty-five, Milliman thought, *well, why not do it again*? But this time Milliman knew the goal was more titanic than before. The difference between eighty and eighty-five in the body and the brain is significant. He also knew that nutrition would be a factor as he struggled with food intake on the eighty-mile run. Then there was the weather to contend with, as conditions were not favorable. The forecast was for heavy rain, high winds, and temperatures in the 50s. But he was determined.

To prepare for his birthday ultra, he consistently ran thirty or forty miles in one day per week, which would take ten hours. He chronicles some of these training runs in his blog. Here is the entry for October 17: "My thirty-mile run Monday started out with my usual thoughts: *Why am I doing this? Ego? Proving something to myself, seeing the challenge to see if my body can hold out at eighty-five years old? Or doing it just because I can?* I did not see an out for myself except for two choices. Stop running or just continue on. By this time I was about seven miles into the run and forgot the arguments with myself and just began to enjoy the beautiful sunrise. The maple leaves turning gold especially in the sunrise were very intense in their color. My first stop at my aid station, home, was 8:30 a.m. Shirley fried me a pancake-egg sandwich, which was excellent! And a cup of hot chocolate. I stopped one more time to change shirts and eat. This was at twenty miles and the time was 12:30. The rest of the training went very well. My training for the past month has been a couple of trail workouts plus my running. One a jogging trail from Deer park, Blue Mt., on Grand Ridge about 8 miles. Good day on that run. Tough steep trail, but I made it."

And another entry on November 4 after a training run: "I have managed my aid by myself. I stop at the house between loops and Shirley makes me a fried egg and bacon bits sandwich. Boy is it good after 5 hours of running. I carry 6 fig bars and 5 dates with me in my camel back so I can run one of my 9-10 mile loops before I have to stop for a refill on my fuel."

On his eighty-fifth birthday, he gathered the same support crew and added additional friends to accompany him along the journey. Shirley was stationed in the motor home and charged with making sure he had hot food and dry clothes. His goal was to finish in thirty hours. This time he began at 10:00 a.m. on his birthday to avoid running through two nights. Here is his account of the event:

"I really felt good until mile 65, twenty to go. And then my back started to tighten up. From then on, it was pain, pain, and more pain. My pit stops to the motor home were getting longer and longer. Everyone was getting concerned. To help with the back pain, my granddaughter Melissa massaged my back and rubbed in menthol, which helped. I was slowing down to a point where I was doing a thirty-seven-minute-per-mile pace. I had been using walking sticks from mile 69 to the end of the race and listing to the right so much that everyone started to worry I wouldn't make the distance. At mile 75 there was an intervention to get me to quit, but that wasn't an option. At about mile 80.5 my friend Larry held my right arm, which took a lot of the pressure off of my back. At my next pit stop my son-in-law Dick came in and read the riot act to me. He said 'I am going to take your other arm and between Larry and me, you are going to do the next four miles without stopping.' He took my right arm and straightened me up. That helped to take the pressure off of my back so that I could walk upright. With that help I managed to walk at about twenty minutes per mile for the last four miles and we were done!"

Not only did he suffer from the physical pain and body breakdowns, but he also struggled to keep his mental side alert, especially during the cold, rainy nights. "At times I thought I would lose my mind out there," recalls Milliman. "I did the multiplication tables, worked on my pace, whatever it took to keep alert and not think about the pain." He finished in thirty-five hours and thirty-five minutes. Along the way he was met with kindness and support from neighbors and friends. One particular act of kindness that still chokes him up was a visit from a 107-year-old neighbor, Larue, who brought him home-baked banana bread at 3:30 in the morning. Her aid drove her to where Milliman was on the course. Larue was his piano teacher when he decided to pick it up at age seventy-four. She was ninety-one at the time.

When asked why he sets such insurmountable goals, he pauses and says, "I'm puzzled by that question myself." He breaks all the stereotypes for his age. You won't find him in a rocking chair any time soon.

Maybe it's his survival instincts that give him the stubbornness of a mule to forge ahead and the determination to succeed against all odds. Maybe it's because he is surrounded by his loved ones, family and friends that he holds close to his heart and who believe in him. Maybe it's because he simply doesn't think like an old man. He thinks he can do anything. While recovering from hernia surgery in 2014, he signed up for a 50K trail run.

Milliman has a strong connectivity to the earth and can get downright spiritual when talking about the Olympic Peninsula where he lives. His blog is filled with postings and pictures about the beauty of its ruggedness, the raw winds, and craggy beaches. He runs in shorts and T-shirts into the winter until his legs turn blue. He worries about his tulips and daffodils when there is a late-spring frost. He marvels at the hummingbird that has taken claim of the feeder in his backyard. His favorite pastime is walking his two Pomeranians on the beach and watching them run with boundless energy, just like their master. He's funny, too. When he runs his usual loop for the umpteenth time and passes the same geese and deer along the way, he imagines that they talk to one another and say, "There he goes again—what a handsome man!"

Milliman talks about aging through the decades and what he has experienced in himself and what he sees at the senior games he attends. During his fifties and sixties, he felt fit and strong and had stiff competition throughout the decade. In his seventies, he noticed the competition dropping off but some were still strong and fighting to the finish. The eighties showed a severe drop not only in numbers of competitors but pace and agility. And now at eighty-five, he struggles to keep a 15:00 pace. "But I'm still out there and feel great," he laughs. "As long as my body can stay upright, I'll compete. I do not run because I must. I do not run for other people. I run because I can. I run for the sheer enjoyment of being able to run. And I thank God every day for my health and that I can still run."

He credits his family and his deep faith with his ability to do what he does. "We all need a support system to get through life and I have the best," says Milliman. He's content. When not running, he tends to his beloved garden, deadheading his dahlias in the fall; he spends time with Shirley, teasing her in the most loving way; he stays in touch with his kids and grandkids; and gives thanks to God every day for a blessed life.

Tom Perri

DOB: June 7, 1961

Residence: Maple Grove, Minnesota

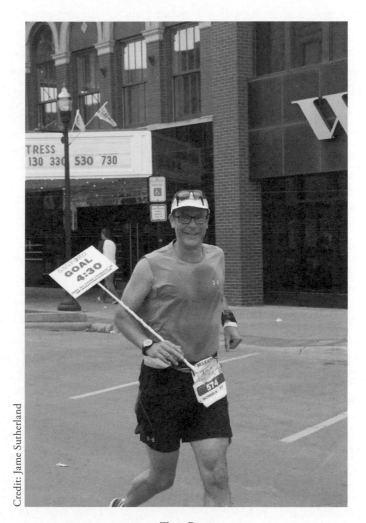

Tom Perri

"Ignore the bumps in the road."

Tom Perri is a triple-time finisher of the 50 States Marathon Club and is already working on the fourth go-round, expected to be completed in 2018. While working on his third-time finish, he also achieved a goal of running all his fifty state marathons in sub-four hours. He'll start again for the fifth tour in 2019. Perri's lifetime running statistics doesn't have one number that isn't a triple digit. His lifetime miles as of May 2018 are 106,209 and that is only going to increase. His two-thousandth career race was completed at Missoula Marathon on July 9, 2017. Despite his most impressive runner statistics and honors, he is most proud of his role as a marathon pacer. "I get more joy out of helping others achieve their goals than out of any of my personal accomplishments," says Perri.

He grew up in Minnesota and describes himself as an outdoorsy kid involved in all sports. He ran track his first two years of high school but switched to band and honors programs by junior year. "I was definitely more the geek than the athlete," he laughs. Graduating high school in 1979, in college he double-majored in English and psychology and then went on to graduate school where he earned two degrees, one in human development and the other in psychology. "I'm a Gemini; I do everything at least twice," he says emphatically.

He picked up running again in his twenties as a social outlet to be with friends. "I didn't grow up wealthy, so my tastes in life tend to be simple," he explains. "Running is cheap. All you need is a T-shirt, a pair of running shoes that don't have to break the bank, and maybe a few bucks for a 5K entry." He ran his first marathon in 1993 at age thirty-two to celebrate both finishing graduate school and his brother's wedding. He attended the Friday night rehearsal dinner, was the best man at the Saturday wedding that went on until 1:30 a.m., and then drove to the start of the Twin Cities Marathon and slept in his car until it was time to take the 5:00 a.m. bus to the start. He had no idea what he was getting himself into. By mile 17 his feet were killing him and bleeding from blood blisters. He walked the last nine miles, finishing in a respectable 3:51. His first reaction was, "One and done. Never doing that again."

That was fourteen years and 419 marathons ago. When I speak with Perri, he is precise, serious, and more than accurate. He can back up all his records. This is his life's work. He never married, retired at forty and dedicates his time to running marathons. He runs an average of forty marathons a year, sometimes putting in a Saturday-Sunday event. He's never had a serious injury that kept him from a marathon. In 2005, he underwent ACL surgery for a torn meniscus that was un-related to running. Thirty-one days later he walked-ran a marathon. "I know my body and how to take care of it," he says about his injury-free running. If he feels a tweak or a ping somewhere, he addresses it imme-diately with a massage or stretching. He runs through an average of five pairs of shoes a year and then donates the used ones. He's a minimalist and doesn't keep anything that isn't of use. He gives most of his medals away to Medals4Mettle, an organization that donates them to children and adults for the mettle and courage they demonstrate battling can-cer, chronic illness, trauma, and other life challenges. In his will, it is stipulated that at his funeral any leftover medals be given to family and friends.

During our interview, Perri and I cover a myriad of topics related to his life on the run. I ask him about the changes he has seen on the circuit since he started in 1993. He doesn't hesitate in responding with the most significant change he has seen: more females on the race circuit. The second biggest change he mentions is technology, as in headphones, Garmin watches, GPS trackers, etc. "It takes the fun out of running," he laments. "With headphones, you don't hear the crowds cheering, which is the best part of the race." And then he rants about the bling factor at races, which is reflected in the race fees. "Why do I have to pay $180 to run a marathon which part of that fee covers the bling cost? I don't care about the swag."

He also talks about how running a marathon in all fifty states has changed as well since he started his quest in 2002. Back then there weren't as many marathons as there are now so the planning was a lot more difficult. For example, in 2005 according to marathonguide.com. there were 314 marathons in the United States, with more than 50 percent taking place in October and November. Today there are more than 1,100 marathons in the United States, according to the latest sta-tistics from the Running USA Annual Marathon report. Perri, being a numbers cruncher, estimated that there are now only twenty-seven days in the calendar where there isn't a marathon.

Perri is taking advantage of all those marathons. After his so-called "one-and-done" marathon in 1993, he came back in 1994 and added Grandma's Marathon to the list along with the Twin Cities Marathon. In 1995, he added the Disney Marathon, bringing his yearly marathons to three. In 2002, he met Steve Boone who, along with his wife Paula, had just started the 50 States Marathon Club. The goal of the group is to run a marathon in all fifty states. Today there are more than four thousand members ranging in age from sixteen to eighty. After meeting Boone, Perri decided to join the club. It took him five years to finish the first tour. "Minnesota is twelve hours from nowhere," he laughs. "To save money, I drove to as many races as I could, sleeping in my car. I tried to squeeze in doubles, running a marathon in Mississippi on a Saturday and then driving to Alabama on Sunday for another." As he made his way through the states, he met other runners on the same quest and became fast friends. They shared tips on how to save money and time when trying to complete the fifty states. "Those people are still my friends today, and we look forward to seeing each other at marathons," says Perri.

Nowadays he is focused on being a pace leader. He is a sought-after pacer, with more than one thousand runners following him to marathons to run with him. Most are looking for a Boston qualifying time, and Perri is the pacer for that. At the 2015 Myrtle Beach Marathon, he brought twelve runners to their BQ time. When I catch up with Perri, he had just finished the Twin Cities Marathon October 1 and then a week later paced the 5:10 group for the 2017 Chicago Marathon. He had one hundred runners in his group, which consisted of four pacers—two in the front, two in the back—and a floater. He was the floater. The following weekend he paced the 4:20 group at the Des Moines Marathon. I ask Perri who started the whole pacing concept and he credited Amby Burfoot. Sure enough, Burfoot confirmed that and says it is one of his legacies he is most proud of, right up there with winning the 1968 Boston Marathon. He told me the story.

In 1995, when he was editor in chief at *Runner's World*, Burfoot was invited out to the St. George Marathon in Utah where thousands of runners were desperately trying to qualify for the one hundredth Boston Marathon the following April. Burfoot got the idea to help the runners qualify by forming pacing groups with his editors, all top runners. He wasn't sure the concept would work but he'd give it a try. Nothing gained, nothing lost. So they promoted the idea and when he went out to do the talk the night before the marathon, he walked on stage to an audience of two thousand interested runners. It was enormously successful with nearly a third of the field getting their coveted BQ. Thus, the pacing concept was born and continues to thrive. Perri is in a select group of pacers who are invited by major marathons such as Chicago and New York City to be pace leaders. And he loves it.

He runs so many marathons that he has legacy at many of them. "I love an inaugural marathon," he claims. "The problem is I feel obligated to return to run them." He's paced the Christie Clinic Illinois Marathon nine straight years and in 2018, it also marked his four-hundredth marathon. When asked about his favorites, he is hard pressed. He loves the Chicks in Charge, the nickname of the female race directors, at the Little Rock Marathon and says that, "they put on a fabulous race." He loves the crowds at the New York City and Chicago Marathons. "You can't beat them for best spectators," he says. He lists Miami as a favorite but mostly because it gets him out of Minnesota in the winter.

Despite all his running, Perri stays injury-free. He underwent ACL surgery in 2005, but that didn't stop him from completing a marathon twenty-eight days later. "I did a walk/run, so that makes it all right," justifies Perri. "I know my body and its limitations." He listens to the tweaks and twinges and then rests and gets a massage. He's not a real advocate of stretching but will do "minimal stretches after a race." His goal is to run 200,000 lifetime miles and believes he can. "I might be eighty, but I'll get there," laughs Perri. I wouldn't bet against him. Perri kicked off 2018 with the Dallas Double, a marathon on Saturday and Sunday. His combined time was 8:02. Starting off 2018, his winter marathon plans were derailed due to blizzards, airport closings and race cancellations. "I missed three marathons due to nor'easters back east," he laments. His luck, and the weather, changed in April. He executed a double marathon weekend that kicked off Thursday, April 26, when he drove five hours to Cedar Rapids, Iowa, spent the night and then on Friday drove four hours to Illinois for the Illinois Marathon on Saturday. He has legacy there, having run it from its inauguration nine years ago and is the only pacer to have paced it every year. He finished in 4:30, then jumped in his car and drove back to Cedar Rapids, Iowa, for the inaugural Cedar Rapids Marathon on Sunday. Welcome to a typical Tom Perri weekend. He's already planned a future goal for his sixtieth birthday. He wants to run six hundred marathons before he turns sixty-one and to BQ in all fifty states.

What can other senior runners learn from Perri? He has a passion for running and for helping others achieve their goals. Running is his life and career. And like any career, he works hard, takes care of himself so he doesn't miss work, and is goal-oriented. No one gives him a raise if he does well. He gets his bonus from the emails that pour in from runners in his pace group. Runners like Michele Prell, who he paced at the 2017 Des Moines Marathon, her first: "Tom was an amazing pacer. Once we got through the crowd during the first three miles, his personality and positivity carried the group through the miles. He was personable, asking questions about each of us. He was concerned, asking other runners if they were okay if they looked like they were struggling, even if they weren't with our group. He was encouraging and did everything he could to get the crowd involved, which made the miles, go by quickly (well, as quickly as 4.5 hours of running can go!). He reminded us to take hills easy and when we needed to push and knew exactly what was coming up on the course to prepare us."

Since Perri is at race events just about every weekend, he has a birds-eye view of the running community and how seniors are playing an increasing larger role. "I really believe that the age of a person is really just a number that in reality has minimal impact on what a person can try to accomplish or achieve in life with running," says Perri. "While I see more and more younger runners at races, I am also seeing more and more runners in the older age groups. Age group awards in the seventies division used to be rare, but now it is becoming rare that there are not runners in their eighties crossing the finish line." The lesson to learn from Perri is to follow your dream down the road and don't let the little bumps get in the way. And more importantly, share the gift of running with others.

Kimi Puntillo

DOB: 1956

Residence: Long Island, NY

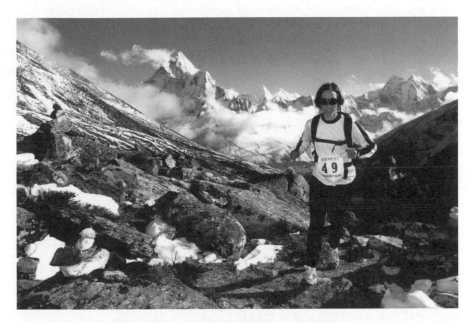

Kimi Puntillo at the Everest Marathon

"Don't waste a day of your life."
Although never a runner, Kimi Puntillo decided to run the 1995 New York City Marathon to help cope with a difficult time in her life. She had watched the marathoners as they ran through Manhattan and always admired their grit and stamina. She took her training seriously and finished, an experience she found beyond thrilling. That marathon changed her

life and she started looking for another race. The Antarctica Marathon, which had been held for the first time earlier that year, appeared on her running radar. "A childhood dream of mine was to go to Antarctica," she says. "I thought, this is my destiny." It became more than a destiny. It became a quest to become the first female to run a marathon on all seven continents. She completed that quest in seven hundred days between 1996 and 1998. Her Guinness Book of World Records entry has since been beaten, but she will always have the honor to be the first.

Puntillo, who grew up in Plandome, Long Island, hated running as a child. "I still remember the Presidential Fitness Test I had to take in high school, a 500-yard dash. I could barely make it around the track. She was good at other sports like field hockey and tennis but never excelled as a runner. After graduating from Tufts, she moved to Washington, DC, to take a job with CBS News, then moved to New York to obtain her MBA and MS in media management from Columbia, settling into the New York City life. In the mid-1990s the New York City running scene was taking off but she still hadn't caught the running bug. She recalls a rainy night and seeing a group of runners training in Central Park. She thought, "Really? In the rain?"

In her mid-thirties, personal setbacks convinced her that she needed to shake up her life. She recalled how inspirational runners in the New York City Marathon were. "I can't think of any other event where the city comes out and is so positive and supportive of so many runners," says Puntillo. "The runners were motivated and full of life. I wanted to feel that." It inspired her to want to run it someday. But when? "I realized that if I don't do it now, it might slip by. Your life gets turned upside down, and you realize that life is short," she says.

She started training for the marathon the same way she approached her work and life in general—by giving it her all and working hard. Every runner she met, she asked for advice. One friend said, "Hitting the Wall is often hyped up, but it's all about the training. If you train well you won't hit the Wall."

The 1995 New York City Marathon was by far the coldest ever. The wind blew at 21 to 32 miles an hour throughout, with gusts on the Verrazano-Narrows Bridge at the start reaching 58 miles per hour, with a wind-chill factor of 18 degrees. Not the best day for a marathon but quite fitting for someone who would run the Antarctica Marathon. Puntillo did well for her first marathon, finishing in 4:34:49, an impressive time for someone who didn't like to run. Her most important lesson was never to say you hate to run, or hate anything for that matter.

Running brought a number of surprises to her life. Never a morning person, the routine of 6:30 a.m. runs changed the time she willingly set her alarm clock. "It was refreshing to rise with the sun and morning runs set a positive tone for the day," she states. It led to becoming athletically fit and paying more attention to what affected her physique. But most importantly she learned not to be intimidated by pushing herself in a new, unchartered direction. "I loved it," she states emphatically.

As a training run for the Antarctic Marathon, she ran the New York City Marathon again in November 1996. By convincing herself to start out slowly and hold back, she took thirteen minutes off her finish time. The following February, she traveled to remote King George Island to fulfill her dream of visiting Antarctica. And it was there that the Guinness record beckoned her to new goals.

The advent of the Antarctica race had made it possible for the first time to run marathons on all seven continents. While on King George Island, Puntillo learned that the first man to accomplish this feat had just been enshrined in the Guinness book. But no woman had done it. "I decided to try to be that woman," she says. On the boat of eighty-nine runners heading to Antarctica she mingled with her fellow explorers. One was a quadriplegic, a young man who was in a drunk driving accident. He was the last to finish, in the dark, while the other runners waited to applaud him. Another was an Aussie who talked about his experience running the Mount Everest Marathon. "I had always wanted to see Mount Everest," she said.

Puntillo already had lined up an assignment to write about her Antarctica experience. Her quest to set a Guinness-sanctioned record generated further assignments. She already had North America completed with the New York City Marathon in 1996. Next up was Europe, completing the London Marathon in April 1997. That was followed by Asia and the Mount Everest Marathon in 1997, then the Mount Kilimanjaro Marathon in June 1998, to check off Africa. Australia's Sydney Marathon was September 1998 and finally the Adidas Marathon in Buenos Aires, October 1998. She crossed the finish line in Buenos Aires one year, eleven months, and one day after she finished the 1996 New York Marathon.

Her toughest marathon out of the seven was Mount Everest in 1977. "It was like running in Heaven but the starting line was at 17,007 feet. The air was so thin that the runners' average marathon finish time was doubled," she recalls. Plus, it took three weeks of trekking to get to the start line.

Running had been so rewarding, she continued to race, even after completing her goal, but suffered a major setback. In 2014 while skiing, another skier ran into her, causing a tear to her ACL. After recovering, she attempted her first post-accident race. Unfortunately, running became much more difficult, and to top it off she came down with food poisoning at the Mongolian Marathon the day before the race. She completed it despite the setbacks because tenacity is what marathon running taught her. Her new goal is to complete one marathon a year.

Puntillo's running brought her not only a place in the records' book, but a globetrotting career as a runner and a journalist, taking her to places as far flung as Bhutan and the North Pole. She parlayed her experiences in a book about adventure runs, titled *Great Races, Incredible Places: 100+ Fantastic Runs Around the World* to share some of the most unique race courses in the world with fellow runners.

Reflecting on her running career, her best advice is: "Get up and try hard every day. Never waste life."

Bill Rodgers

DOB: December 31, 1947

Residence: Boxborough, Massachusetts

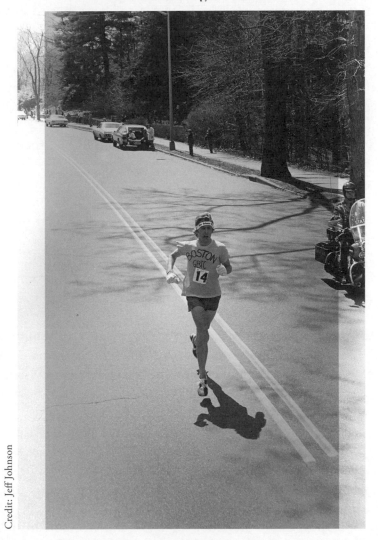

Credit: Jeff Johnson

Bill Rodgers

"I never met a runner I didn't like."

Bill Rodgers, best known for his victories in the Boston and New York City marathons in the late 1970s, winning both four times, twice breaking the American record at Boston with a time of 2:09:55 in 1975, an American and course record and a 2:09:27 in 1979, is a running legend. At the height of his career he was one the most-recognized and beloved marathoner in the country. In 1977, he became the first person in history to simultaneously hold the Boston, New York City, and Fukuoka marathon titles and remains the only person to have achieved this feat.

By the end of his competitive career at age forty, he had run fifty marathons, twenty-nine of them under 2:15. In 2008, he was diagnosed with prostate cancer, which caught him by surprise. But nothing stops Boston Billy, and he came back stronger and healthier after beating it. Rodgers continues to connect with runners around the world with his charm, stories, and passion for the sport.

Rodgers was born in Hartford, Connecticut. His best friends were his older brother, Charlie, and their friend Jason. The trio did everything together, running like a pack of puppies around the neighborhood. In high school they put their running to good use, joining the cross-country team where Rodgers excelled. "I loved it from the start," he recalls. "I loved the open territory and going the distance." On the other hand, he was not good at track, saying he lacked the initial kick required for short distances. His talent was noticed and on Mondays he often enjoyed hearing his name on the principal's PA system announcing the athlete of the week.

At Wesleyan University he continued to run cross country but slacked off a bit, enjoying the college life. His roommate, Amby Burfoot, was a standout runner also from Connecticut. When Burfoot returned to their room after one weekend, it was strewn with beer cans and cigarette butts. One Sunday morning not long after, Burfoot took Rodgers on a twenty-five-mile run. "I think he was getting back at me for the beer cans," laughs Rodgers. "I kept up pretty well 'til the end when Amby picked up the pace and dropped me." What Rodgers may not have known then was that Burfoot was seriously thinking about a Boston Marathon win. Burfoot's high school coach, John J. Kelley, won the Boston Marathon in 1957 and Burfoot dreamed of doing the same. One weekend Kelley came down to Wesleyan and they all went for a long run. Rodgers recalls thinking, "That Kelley guy can run pretty fast for an old man." At the time Kelley was probably thirty-nine. Burfoot went on to win the 1968 Boston Marathon his senior year, in 2:22:17. Rodgers hadn't caught the marathon bug just yet, describing it as too far, too much training. "I thought I'd die if I had to train for a marathon," he tells me.

Rodgers went through a lost period after college. He stopped running, smoked more than the occasional cigarette, couldn't get a job, and had the Vietnam War looming over his head. He received a conscientious objector status for his Roman Catholic beliefs against the war and finally got a job at Peter Bent Brigham Hospital in Boston wheeling bodies to the morgue. He bought a motorcycle with his paycheck. But things got worse. He lost that job and his motorcycle was stolen. He had to now walk or run everywhere, which made him stop smoking.

In April of 1971, he watched the Boston Marathon for the first time. He saw his Wesleyan cross country teammate Jeff Galloway run by along with John Vitale, whom he ran against in college. He thought, if they can run a marathon, so can I. That epiphany changed the course of his life. In 1975, 1977, and 1979, Track & Field News ranked Rodgers number one in the world in the marathon. In all, he won twenty-two marathons in his career. His first attempt at Boston was in 1973, and after putting in 130 miles a week in training, he thought he was poised for somewhere in the top five finishers. But as he was fond of saying later on, the marathon will humble you. He dropped out at mile 21.

Missing the camaraderie and support of his collegiate running days, he joined the Greater Boston Track Club that had just formed. He ran Boston again in 1974, finishing in 14th place in 2:19. His top competitors included Galloway, Tom Fleming, and Jerome Drayton. He recalls Fleming as the fiercest trainer. Fleming was poised to win in '74 but sprained his ankle the Thursday before the marathon. As Tom Derderian writes in his bible of a book, *Boston Marathon*, "There it went. All that preparation (a year's worth of 100-plus miles week) gone to a New Jersey pothole."

Rodgers was hell-bent on winning in 1975. Fresh off his third-place finish at the World Cross Country championships in Rabat, Morocco, he knew he could do it. The press still took him for a lighthearted goof-ball, not a serious contender. And that was fine with Rodgers. "They underestimated my desire to win," he says. "I prayed for the perfect day and my prayers were answered." He went like a bat out of hell and never stopped. He wore a hand-painted Greater Boston Track Club T-shirt, white gardening gloves, a headband given to him by Fleming at the start to hold back his unruly mane of blonde hair, and running shoes borrowed from Steve Prefontaine, which he had to stop and re-tie along the course. He set an American and course record that day in 2:09:55. He was on fire.

In 1976, Fred Lebow invited him to run the first five-borough New York City Marathon. Lebow, always the showman, also invited Frank Shorter and thought the hype of having the Olympic gold medalist and the American record winner from Boston run against each other would be great for his marathon. Rodgers recalls that day: "I didn't even know the course. I remember running on the East Drive promenade passing fisherman and drunks. I loved the New York crowd and fed off their energy." He won in 2:10:10. And in typical Rodgers fashion, he forgot his running shorts and had borrowed a pair of soccer shorts at the last minute. When he finished the race, his car, which had been illegally parked, was towed. Lebow had to take up a collection to get Rodgers's car back.

Rodgers became the most recognizable marathoner in the world. With his boyish face, underdog mentality, and shaggy blond hair, he was a rebel. He was hoping for a berth on the 1980 Olympic marathon team when the United States boycotted the Moscow Olympics. Sixty-eight other countries followed. Rodgers was angry, and the only way he knew to deal with his anger was to run and win his fourth Boston Marathon. But the win didn't come easy. As Derderian recalls in *Boston Marathon*, Rodgers wanted to show his anger to the world and wear a black armband in protest of the boycott. When word of his intentions got out, a death threat came in by phone to his running store. "The anonymous caller warned that Rodgers would not make it alive past Coolidge Corner," writes Derderian. Rodgers backed off. He ran the 1984 Olympic Trials marathon and finished eighth in a time of 2:13:30. Alberto Salazar was primed to win the Trials race, but he placed second to the relatively unknown Pete Pfitzinger, who beat him by one second in 2:11:43. Pfitzinger went on to finish eleventh at the Olympics.

At the beginning of his career, Rodgers never made the big cash that athletes do today. He ran during the era when runners had to be amateurs. In 1976, he didn't have the spare money to drive to New York City on toll roads and took back roads instead. This inequality infuriated Rodgers, who was one of the first runners to challenge the

AAU on their stand against payment for amateurs. He asked Lebow for two thousand dollars under the table to run New York and Lebow paid him out of pocket. In contrast, the 2017 male and female winners at the New York City marathon won $100,000. But all this changed and by 1981 Rodgers was earning appearance money as well as prize money. Gone were his days of living on food stamps and sleeping on mattresses in friends' apartments.

In December of 2007, Rodgers was at a 10K event in Barbados when he got a call from his doctor with bad news: he had prostate cancer. Shocked with the news, he went on to win the 10K and then flew home for surgery in January of 2008. He came back to running, sometimes clocking faster times than before his diagnosis. He also became an advocate for prostate cancer research and early screening. He never talked about retiring but slowed down both in pace and his number of races. "Nowadays I only run in one gear," says Rodgers. "I can't shift into surges or kicks. I think of myself as a dependable car with one steady gear." He attends on average forty races and clinics a year, spending time at expos talking to his fans. He ran an Anniversary Tour in 2015 to celebrate forty years of running, going back to races he won in his heyday like the Cherry Blossom Ten Mile in Washington, DC, the Boilermaker 15K Road Race in Utica, New York, the Falmouth Road Race in Massachusetts, and the Azalea Trail Run in Mobile, Alabama. "Going back to these races is mind-blowing for me," says Rodgers. "I'm not that young guy who won them and the races have grown so much since I ran them." Promoting the sport and mingling with his fans is his main occupation. He last ran the Boston Marathon in 2009, a year after being diagnosed with the cancer. He wore a singlet that supported prostrate cancer and he blended in with the other runners. "No one knew who I was and that was fine with me," says Rodgers, who also supports melanoma research. "Runners are the best fundraisers and if I can help I am more than happy to support a good cause." Even though he doesn't run the marathon anymore he is always out there on race day talking to the runners and the spectators who still can't get enough of "Boston Billy."

At his speaking engagements, he attracts crowds both young and old. The elder runners still revere him as one of them and the younger ones want to beat him. It's not unusual at races for young guns to try and beat him and then boast that they do. He tells me he's okay with it but he still gets competitive and tries to keep up. "I'm still going to try if I can," he laughs. "I want them to beat me. Heck, if they can't beat a geezer, then they have a problem."

Now seventy, Rodgers is stoic and philosophical about his life. "Turning seventy is definitely a challenge," he says. "I'm not going to lie. This feels like an epic age." He's gone from eating junk food to healthy food with an occasional chocolate chip cookie. He's cut back his mileage to forty a week and only runs fifteen races a year. Once famous for double workouts, he now laughs that his second workout of the day is walking his dog. He's into yoga. He thinks about his mortality. He loves seeing that scientific data now supports what he and other runners always believed back in the seventies, that running is good for you. "My entire running life people would say to me, 'What about your knees?' 'What about your feet?' Or my favorite, 'What are you running from?'" Now we are seeing proof that running doesn't affect knees at all and in general keeps us healthy and engaged. He can get philosophical about the aging process and how it is linked to his running: "When I was trying to get into marathon racing, there weren't that many older people out there," Rodgers said. "There are so many really good older runners today and that's a huge change in the sport and shows you the longevity of our sport. The old runners want to keep going. It's the most underrated sport for what it does for your heath and well-being. If you get out the door and stay active, life is better. The evidence of that is clear."

His advice to older runners is simple: "You have to know when to back off. I raced too much and I felt old at forty. I was motivated to win. It's a powerful drug that can also derail a career too early." Nowadays, the crowds he speaks to at race events and meeting new runners motivate him. "I love giving back to this sport that has given me so much," says an older and more subdued Rodgers.

Ed Rousseau

DOB: September 19, 1939

Residence: Minneapolis, Minnesota

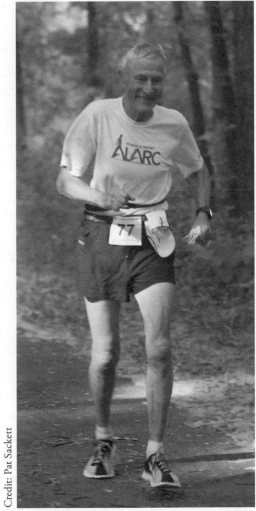

Ed Rousseau

"The longer the race the better."

Ed Rousseau of Minneapolis has run 104 marathons, 113 ultramarathons, and loves races with "hours" in the title, as in a twenty-four-hour race, seventy-two-hour race, and then there are the "day" races he looks forward to, as in the six-day race he ran totaling 384 miles. "A guy's got to run or head for a recliner," explained Rousseau, seventy-eight, in his usual self-effacing manner. "I'll take running." What he is most proud of though, despite his numerous age-group records, is his thirty-four years of sobriety.

Rousseau came into this world literally in a shoebox. Born in the sticks of upper Michigan in a town with a population of one hundred, he came early, at seven months, weighing only three pounds. A creative nurse at the local hospital put him in a shoebox and attached a light bulb to it to simulate an incubator to keep him alive. Her method worked and Rousseau grew up on his parents' farm doing chores, running cows, and learning to hunt, trap, and love the outdoors. His parents instilled in him a strong work ethic early in life. Besides his farm chores, he had to earn his spending money during the summers by peeling the bark off logs. Paper mills were a big industry back then and the loggers needed to strip the bark off the logs before they would accept them at the mill. Kids like Rousseau were hired to strip the bark for three cents a log. Starting at twelve years old, he would head into the woods with a sharp metal tool he made himself to strip the bark. The hardest part of the job was dealing with the insects that plagued the workers. There was no insect repellent back then so Rousseau's father made his own batch mixing kerosene with pine tar and then lined his hat with it to repel the flies and bugs. It worked, but the odor was so bad it made him sick. "I would vomit from the smell, but I didn't get any bug bites," laughs Rousseau. "That would probably be child abuse these days."

The only sport his high school offered was basketball. With winter lasting about nine months, there were no baseball or track and field events. His team was highly successful, winning two state championships. He still can recall the championship game played at Michigan State University's field house in front of twelve thousand people. "It was an education just to play there," recalls Rousseau.

After high school, he didn't want to go the normal route of most of the kids in town and become a logger. "I liked my toes and fingers too much!" he laughs. At seventeen, he enlisted in the Air Force. During basic training, he had to run three miles on a track. His basketball years prepared him for endurance running and also with a desire to win: "I was not going to be last. I was going to win." He finished his first three-mile run out front and realized he was a good runner. Although the Air Force was a good move for him career-wise, he started drinking on a regular basis. Alcoholism runs in his family and he became its next victim. Beer was his best buddy.

After he left the Air Force, Rousseau worked on technology projects for a data corporation and was sent to Tehran. He loved Iran, learned to speak the language and found a way to continue his drinking. A co-worker lived a mile up the hill from him and they would meet there to play cribbage and drink beer. During the fall of 1978, right before the coup, the Iranian military issued a nighttime curfew of 9:00 p.m. You had to be off the streets or risk getting shot. At 8:45, Rousseau would sprint the mile back to his apartment, just avoiding the bullets. "My running came in handy," he laughs. "It enabled me to have one more game and one more beer." He drank steadily while in Iran. He recalls the 1978 New Year's Eve party at the Sheraton ballroom. No one could leave due to the curfew so the party went on until 5:00 in the morning. When the revolution was in full swing, he returned to the States in 1979.

Back home, his drinking continued. It cost him his marriage and one too many DUIs. He recalls going before a judge who could have sentenced him to time in jail but instead read him the riot act. It made an impression on Rousseau and he started going to AA. "I had to face the fact that my so-called social drinking was a serious problem," he says. Years later when that judge died, Rousseau read his obituary. Turns out the judge was a former alcoholic and felt that the best way to handle those cases was to get the person in treatment. Rousseau took his AA counseling seriously at first and combined it with his running. Although he kept up running in Iran, it was only quick sprints, about a mile at a time at most. During the five years he was in Iran, the running boom in the United States had taken hold, fueled by Frank Shorter's 1972 Olympic gold medal in the marathon. Rousseau saw people out jogging, something new to him. At age forty, he decided to join them and pulled on his old sweat pants, twenty-year-old basketball shoes, and went for a run. He barely made it around the block. His deteriorating health from alcoholism and shortness of breath from years of smoking took its toll. It was also his wake-up call.

He kept it up, running a bit farther with each new day. He lost the beer gut and stayed sober. Says Rousseau of those enlightening days: "I replaced the high of running with the high of getting drunk." He remarried, increased his mileage and started entering races. Things were looking up in his life until Thanksgiving, one year into his sobriety. He participated in a family toast and kept toasting. His sobriety was over. In retrospect, he admits to not keeping up with the AA meetings or at the very least reinforcing the improvement steps he had learned. Even though he was back to drinking, he kept up his running and racing and eating healthy. He didn't gain back the beer belly and in fact, his racing times were never better. Says Rousseau of this period, "I raced to get rid of the hangover."

After numerous drinking and driving incidents, he swore off drinking for the second time. And this time, it stuck. He's been sober for thirty-four years. "I work every day at being sober," says a reformed Rousseau. "My creed is, 'I have alcoholism. It is a disease with no cure so I run instead of drinking.'"

During his second stint at sobriety, he ran every day. One day while out running he met a fellow runner who asked him if he was going to run the new marathon. "I had heard of Boston but didn't realize there were other ones," laughs Rousseau. He and his new friend signed up for the inaugural Twin Cities Marathon in 1982. He was forty-three at the time. He kept going back and he is now one of only twenty-three left of the charter members and the oldest one. His dream is to run the fiftieth consecutive Twin Cities Marathon at age ninety-two. I wouldn't bet against him to be there.

Two years later he ran his first Boston Marathon and two years after that he ran his first ultra, the Edmund Fitz 100K. He kept looking for more challenges and started running races of twelve hours, twenty-four hours, and just about every distance including a six-day race. He won his first one-hundred-miler in his late forties. "My legs hurt so bad during that one I didn't think I would finish but I knew someone was right behind me so the competitive juices kicked in and I started sprinting," recalls Rousseau, who finished in nineteen hours. A week later he ended up in the hospital with total kidney failure. Turns out his muscles were so depleted they started eating his body's protein sources. On top of that he started taking ibuprofen for the pain. The combination overwhelmed the kidneys and they shut down. By the time he was in the hospital, his creatinine levels, which should be one milligram in a male, were over seven. His doctor warned him he might be facing dialysis for life. Fortunately for Rousseau his kidneys kicked in a few days later. He's never taken ibuprofen again. But he keeps running ultras.

His next ultra was the FANS 24 Hour Ultra Running Race in Minneapolis. FANS, which stands for "Furthering Achievement through a Network of Support," supports urban teenagers in achieving their goal of earning a college education. The course is a 2.14-mile loop around a lake. He took second with 110 miles. He loves that event and has done it for thirty years straight. His personal best for that event is 121 miles.

He has suffered his share of injuries and contributes them to over-exuberance and over-training. He stopped running so-called "junk miles" and now runs about thirty miles a week. He runs maintenance miles twice a week, has one day for speed work, takes three rest days and then one long run up to thirty miles. He eats healthy, follows the food pyramid ("thank God alcohol isn't part of the pyramid," he adds), and cross trains. In the winter he'll put on some wooden snowshoes and head into the woods by his cabin. He has started a walk-run routine for his ultras, which helps with the injuries, and he found he didn't lose any time. He still bites off more than he can chew as he did in September of 2017. He entered the 24-Hour Nationals in Cleveland where he won his age division and then two weeks later ran his thirty-first consecutive Twin Cities Marathon.

He is very pragmatic about his loss of speed over the years. At seventy-eight, his best times are definitely in the past but he doesn't dwell on it. His best marathon time was 2:57 in 1984 at age forty-five and he just ran Twin Cities in 5:10. His best mileage for a twenty-four-hour race is 121 at fifty-four and at the nationals he ran eighty-three miles. "I just stay competitive in my age division and that's challenging enough for me," he says. "I am finally getting smart and using my semblance of a brain when it comes to my running."

When asked why he kept raising the bar, he laughs: "Instead of another drink I run another mile." Realizing he will always be a recovering alcoholic with an addictive personality, he needs to keep looking for new adventures. Despite his athletic achievements, what makes him stand out is his empathy for others, especially other alcoholics. He volunteers at AA meetings and other treatment centers as a motivational speaker. He goes to county jails and speaks to the inmates about addiction. His favorite line is, "Maybe you can handle that one glass. It's the next ten that get you in trouble." He lives by the motto, "be the best you can be." He's very aware of the pitfalls of falling off the wagon and feels that by engaging in motivational talks he is also helping himself. "If I don't give back I may fall back," he reminds himself. He's learned to handle the bad with the good and considers himself very lucky. He's healthy, successful in his second marriage, and loves his running life.

He recently attended his sixtieth high school reunion back in that logger town in the upper peninsula of Michigan. The alumni group is now down to ten. He had a shock when his best friend from high school that he always looks forward to seeing died a week before the reunion from brain cancer. "I had to go to extra AA meetings to help me get through that emotional crisis," he says. At the reunion, his classmates weren't in great shape. One was on oxygen from a lifetime of smoking. Others were limping, out of shape, grumpy. "I'm in great shape for the shape I'm in!" he laughs.

Rousseau gets philosophical when I ask him about his future. He describes his running as a lifesaving tool that has the bonus of providing him with a group of close-knit people who are like family to him, even though he may only see them once a year at a race. "I look forward to going to events because it's like a family reunion," he says. "We all train and push to be our competitive best but yet we are humble and friendly on a personal level." It reminds him of a quote from Arnold Palmer: "It's much more important to be nice." He relies on his faith to be the best person he can be. Rousseau sums up his ideology: "Like all areas of life; we are here to learn, grow, and improve on a daily basis."

With his thirty-four-year sobriety medal tucked in the back pocket of his pants as a daily reminder of his commitment, Rousseau has a lot of wisdom, which he is happy to share with anyone who needs a friend.

Alan Ruben

DOB: March 9, 1957

Residence: Manhattan, New York

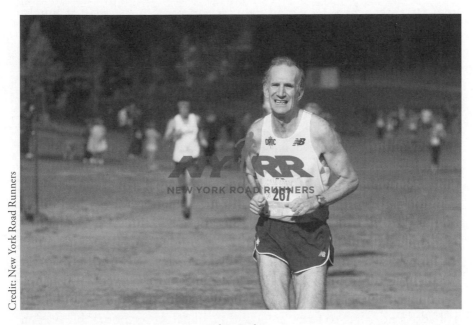

Alan Ruben

"How fast can I run?"

Soft-spoken, with a British reserve that hides a competitive nature, Alan Ruben is part of the fabric of an elite group of runners in New York. He has run every New York City Marathon since 1987 and for twenty-five years, from 1989 to 2014, he kept a sub-3:00 streak. He is dedicated to his training with Central Park Track Club where he has been a member for twenty-eight years. Through his thirty-three years of running, he has perfected his stride and pacing and uses those skills to pass unsuspecting rivals with patience and persistence. Everything in Ruben's life, his family, work, and running, was at a pinnacle until 2015 when he suffered a mild stroke. But with stoicism and resolve, he ran the marathon eight months after the diagnosis in 4:28:24. It was far from his fastest but it was his most gratifying. Getting back on track was slow going, but Ruben is relentless. He ran the 2017 New York City Marathon, two years after the stroke, in 3:12:41 at age sixty.

Ruben was born in London, England. His high school was close to Regent's Park, where he would play pickup soccer every day at lunchtime. Organized sports at school were rugby and cricket. On days when it was too wet to play rugby, his class ran a two-mile cross-country course. That was his introduction to running. He occasionally ran races against other schools and enjoyed it. He came in second in his school's ninth-grade cross-country race. The following year he came back determined to win, and he did. "I still have that certificate," says Ruben with a smile.

At Manchester University, where he majored in math, sports took a back seat to socializing. When he graduated in 1978 he took a job with a computer company. He settled into a post-collegiate life of work and meeting friends afterward. In 1983, encouraged by friends who were running the London Marathon he signed up for the lottery and started training, but when he got rejected he stopped running. He reapplied for the next two years but never got in and switched his focus to the 1985 Paris Marathon. His training for a first marathon was underwhelming. He ran one long run of two hours, raced a half marathon, and thought he had it in the bag to meet his goal time of sub-three hours. He was on pace for the first half but then crashed and burned during the second half. "I just wanted to finish this silly thing and never have to do another," says Ruben. "This was definitely a one and done." He finished in 3:09:53, an excellent time for a first marathon despite Ruben's "crash-and-burn" description of his run. Ruben's competitive nature started early in his marathon career.

One month later he was transferred to New York. The next time he ran was in the Corporate Challenge. After that he started running regularly again. After two years in Manhattan his assignment was coming to an end. Before he left he decided to run the New York City Marathon as a way of saying goodbye to the city he had come to love.

He ran the 1987 New York City Marathon in 3:00:37, but still wasn't satisfied with his time.

Back in Europe, he ran the 1988 Dublin Marathon in 2:59:18, finally breaking three hours. A week later, back in New York, he ran the New York City Marathon in 3:01:57. Motivated by his fast times, he finally got into the London Marathon and ran 2:47:45 and then ran Berlin in 2:39:28. His running career started to take off. "I wanted to get more serious and competitive with my running," says Ruben. "I was motivated and loved the feeling." After his two-year return to London, he settled permanently in New York in October of 1990. The Manhattan running scene not only gained a new rising star, a New York City Marathon streak was born.

In 1990, after a race in Central Park, he met a runner from Central Park Track Club who encouraged him to join. And as he says with a sly smile, "the rest is history." His running took off. "I ran with great runners, had a great coach, and loved working hard." Not only did his running improve, he met his future wife, Gordon Bakoulis. "I knew of her before I met her," he recalls. "She won all the races and I tried my hardest to beat her."

Ruben was dedicated to his training. Nothing was hard or fast enough for him. At the 1998 Boston Marathon he ran his lifetime PR, 2:29:54, nine months after the birth of his first son. The years and the marathons flew by. He motored along with patience and persistence, a fine-tuned running machine. If he felt an injury coming on he addressed it right away. He's a smart runner who knows his limits even as he keeps pushing them. His marathon training rarely went beyond ninety miles a week. He was able to find that balance between wanting to improve and at the same time being cautious. This worked well for him through his forties. Pushing into his fifties, he admits that "running just got harder."

Despite his British reserve and stiff-upper-lip first impression, Ruben has a dry sense of humor. He is a family man first and loves nothing more than spending time with his wife and three boys. On his Central Park Track Club home page, which goes back to the late 1990s, his wit is often employed. Friends' humorous digs on this page make it clear that Ruben is beloved by all. He is teased about being in just about every piece of televised footage of the New York City Marathon. There's Alan, up front with the professional women. There's Alan again, entering Central

Park. There's Alan on the heels of Franca Fiacconi, third-place female finisher in the 1997 race. One friend posted about being in Europe on vacation and watching the television and, yes, seeing Alan running the New York City Marathon. "Get that man off my television screen," posted his friend. "He's everywhere!" But when you win or place in just about every race you run and have won the New York Road Runners prestigious Runner of the Year award seven times, it's hard not to be seen everywhere. In his dry, humorous way, he sums up why he runs: "It just makes me feel better," he says, "and I feel my best when the race is over!"

Fast-forward to March of 2015. Ruben woke up and felt some numbness at the side of his mouth but went about his day. Later that night he was unsteady on his feet and had to hold on to walls for balance. By the next morning the numbness had traveled down the entire right side of his body. He went to a doctor, who ordered a brain scan. Two weeks later he learned he had a mild stroke. Because he is so fit, the doctors were a bit perplexed. Blood tests revealed that he was deficient in the naturally occurring proteins C and S, which serve as anticoagulants. This meant that Ruben's blood was more likely to clot. Whether this led to the stroke is uncertain, but the finding was significant, and he now takes two baby aspirin a day.

By now he was able to walk fairly normally, so, naturally, he tried to run. He was able to run a mile in eleven minutes, and over the next few weeks he got the time down to eight minutes. He resumed training with CPTC in a slower group, despite continuing numbness in his foot. He ran a few races just two minutes off his pre-stroke times, but by August he had developed a severe case of plantar fasciitis. "Because of the numbness, I didn't feel the pain," says Ruben, who would have backed off immediately if he had had any inkling of the injury. He had to stop running for two months to let his foot heal. In October, he did a few test runs and felt better. Determined to preserve his marathon streak, he decided to run the 2015 New York City Marathon—number twenty-eight—even if it meant walking some of the course. In the three weeks leading up to the marathon, his longest run was four miles.

He targeted 3:30 as his goal, but by mile 17 he had to stop and walk. He did a run/walk for the remainder and finished in 4:28:24. He reflects on his slowest marathon: "In some ways it was nice not to run by time and just enjoy the race and the runners and the course. I could feel the crowd support and pick out people I knew along the way." But that feeling of "just enjoying the run" didn't last. The following year he was back in form, running a 3:12:58—and yes, he was disappointed with that.

In his late fifties he began to feel that the training and the workouts were getting tougher, and he started to lose his motivation to run. His times were getting slower; he was never satisfied. "Once I got slower, it became harder to keep up my level of training," he admits. But something big was looming over him in 2017—his thirtieth consecutive New York City Marathon. His year wasn't going well as his times slowed and he worried about struggling through the marathon. "I was motivated to run it, but genuinely unsure if I would continue after that," says Ruben. The marathon did go well and he felt comfortable, running faster than expected. He ran 3:12:41, a few seconds quicker than his 2016 time. "That rejuvenated me, and I will certainly run it in 2018 and probably well beyond," says Ruben. "It showed me it was still possible to enjoy the whole marathon." He quotes a line from the movie *Without Limits* to sum up his feeling on running: "If you can find meaning in this senseless activity of running, maybe you can find meaning in that other meaningless thing—life." Ruben has found that his passion, this "senseless activity," gives meaning to his life.

"My main motivation for running is that it makes me feel better both physically and mentally on a day-to-day basis. Being quite good at it means it is more enjoyable because I do well competitively," he explains. But what happens when the competition gets too tough? When the workouts aren't working? When the younger guys pass him? If his enjoyment of running is tied to speed and winning, can he sustain it as he slows down?

"My motivation is dropping because competitively I have fallen back, say 78 percent age-graded versus 84 percent age-graded previously," he says. He thinks this is due to the stroke. At sixty, he has thoughts about continuing to run but retiring from racing. He actually entertains the thought of no longer doing more hard workouts and less-taxing training runs. But he worries that without the goal of racing as fast as he can in his age division, he'll lose a lot of the motivation. After a bit of reflection, he also realizes that "I would also lose out on the most important benefits of running for me—that it makes me feel better both mentally and physically on a day-to-day basis."

Other age-division aces in Ruben's age group shouldn't consider Ruben out of the running. That competitive streak won't let him stop.

It will also mean that his wife might beat him in every race. He is already planning his thirty-first New York City Marathon. "As long as I have a good time running—and a good time [he says with emphasis], I'll keep going." He looks ahead to his seventies: "I would like to keep running at any level I'm capable of," he says. To get there, he needs to incorporate more strength training and be more conscious of his form—head up, not down. Like most aging runners, he worries about falling. "I know I'll have to be more cautious and sensible as I age," says Ruben. And like most aging runners, he hates to see videos of himself running: "My form is awful, I'm so slow, oh my God, this can't be me!"

With two of the boys in college and one in high school, Ruben and Bakoulis are on their way to being empty-nesters. That could mean more time to run for enjoyment. It could also mean more time for workouts and training. Only Ruben knows what direction he will take when he comes to the fork in the road race. As for now, he flashes a smile and says, with that dry British reserve, "It's been quite nice so far."

Drew Swiss

DOB: November 4, 1957

Residence: Armonk, New York

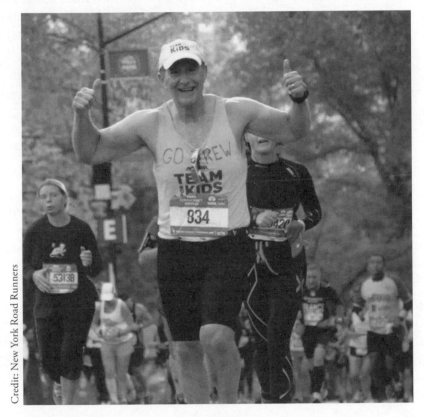

Drew Swiss

"Running is the fountain of youth."

Growing up in hardscrabble household, Drew Swiss had to fight his way through middle school and tolerate bullying for being a chubby kid. He found running as a way to change his life and get fit, and he developed a passion for the sport. By the time he was forty, he had run sixteen marathons and took a break when he started having kids. In 2007, he found a new passion—running for charity. Since finding Team for Kids (TFK), Swiss has dedicated his marathons and half marathons to raising money for this New York Road Runners–sponsored charity for adult runners who sign up to run the New York City Marathon. Funds raised by TFK support running-based fitness, goal-setting, and nutrition programs in underserved schools and communities across the United States. Swiss has been the top fundraiser for ten years, raising more than $700,000 for underserved kids in the program. In 2017, he ran his thirty-second marathon overall and celebrated turning sixty the day after running the New York City Marathon.

Swiss was born in Brooklyn in the Glenwood Projects, a public-housing apartment complex with lots of nearby parks. He was always outside, playing pickup games with his friends. Softball was a religion for the boys. He also had a cerebral side, and he played chess with his friend. "It was a great place to grow up," recalls Swiss. "We had everything we needed in the streets and parks, which were filled with all sorts of characters, all shapes, sizes, and ethnicity."

Although Swiss was happy with his friends in the street, his home life was a struggle. Money was tight and his mother made do with food, reusing Crisco to fry just about everything. "I was a chubby kid with bad eating habits," says Swiss. He wanted a better life, and as early as eight years old he was earning his own money at various jobs, learning responsibility, and how to manage money. He shoveled snow, bussed tables, bagged groceries, and worked at a gas station, and soon he opened his own bank account. At fifteen, he and a friend got jobs pulling rusty spikes from train tracks with a pickaxe and were paid $10 an hour for the dirty, backbreaking work. Says Swiss, "We thought we were rich!" In high school, he got into sports and joined the wrestling team, becoming captain. He also joined the track team, his introduction to running. He started losing weight and got into great shape.

After graduating from high school he was accepted to Brooklyn College, but his father refused to pay the tuition. Swiss knew he was at a pivotal junction in life: move forward with college or stay home with the probability of staying a street kid with a dubious future. He made the decision to move out of the house and get his own apartment. He took numerous part-time jobs to pay for college and his living expenses. He looks back on this as one of the best decisions he ever made in life. He ran everywhere, cooked his own healthy meals, and worked hard at school and his jobs, one of which was driving a tow truck. He was always strapped for cash, but he had his independence. There was nothing Swiss wouldn't do to reach his goal of graduating from college and getting on with his life.

After graduating, he worked at the accounting firm Ernst & Whinney. He was in the best shape of his life and excited about his future. His running increased to fifteen miles a day at times. He was in love with running and with life, excited about all the possibilities. In 1987, the New York City Marathon fell on his thirtieth birthday and he decided to run it. He didn't train well, didn't even have a plan, only putting in one long run of twenty miles. By mile 23 he had severe blisters and had to have his feet wrapped at a medical station. Hoping for a sub-four-hour finish, he completed the marathon in 4:45:35. Frustrated with his time, he joined a training program and his times got faster. He consistently broke four hours in his marathons, running two a year. He got his marathon personal best down to 3:31.

In 1997, Swiss had another life-changing event: at age forty, he got married. Two years later, he and his wife, Amy, had the first of their four kids. His marathons took a backseat to being a father and his then demanding job as vice president of finance for Montefiore Health System in Bronx, Rockland, and Orange Counties, New York. In 2007, he decided to come back to his favorite pastime, running marathons. Now pushing fifty, he found he was slower and got discouraged. Maybe his marathon days were over. He looked with longing to his days of running sub-four-hour marathons, training seventy miles a week, and never being injured. At forty-nine, he was pushing a double baby jogger and wondering if he would ever get back to his former self.

His fiftieth birthday happened to fall on the day of the 2007 New York City Marathon. Planning ahead, his wife Amy asked him if there was anything he would like to do for this milestone event. He said, "The only thing I want is to run the New York City Marathon again." He hadn't run a marathon in eight years and wanted to run it smart, with good training and coaching. He also wanted to run it for a good cause. He started scrolling the list of charity partners for the marathon and stopped when he read the mission statement for TFK. "I instantly related to what they were doing because when I was a kid my mother fed me the worst kinds of food and as a result I had weight issues," says Swiss. "It just resonated with me, so I made it my birthday gift to these kids." With TFK, Swiss found coaches who worked with him to improve his times. He also found a community of runners who, like him, loved the New York City Marathon and running for the cause. He became a fundraising machine, dedicated to raising as much money as he could for the kids. Says Swiss, "The main focus is to get these kids healthy and avoid the most expensive health-care costs in the country that are related to obesity-related illnesses."

In his ten years with TFK, Swiss has raised more than $700,000, all from individual donors. In one year alone he raised $100,000. He does his fundraising the old-fashioned way, sending out personal emails to every single person he has a connection with. Thousands of emails go out, and thousands of people respond and donate. No one escapes Swiss. "When you feel passionate about something, like I do for these kids, it's easy to ask for donations," he says. When an article about his fundraising appeared in his local paper, he told his then nine-year-old son that, "It is important to help others when you are in a position to do so." His son then gave him a dollar and said, "I want to help." Fundraising became a family affair.

What keeps Swiss running after more than forty-five years? Why does he continue to train and push himself? "Running is the most natural thing in the world. It's like breathing to me; I can't live without it," he explains. He's had life-changing experiences while running, such as at the 2013 Boston Marathon, which he ran for charity. He had reached mile 25 when he was stopped, like so many other runners, not realizing what had happened. "The bombing was a tragedy. I will never forget that day," recalls Swiss. But he also remembers the kindness of the Bostonians and how the incident brought out the best in people.

Swiss loves the marathon. "It's an indelible experience, so beautiful to me," he says. "And I am always trying to better my time, so I never get tired of putting in the effort." He's met cool people like Olympian Meb Keflezighi and Paralympian Tatyana McFadden. And he's become a legend at New York Road Runners (NYRR) who own the Team for Kids charity program. Michael Rodgers, NYRR's vice president of development and philanthropy, has this to say about Swiss: "Drew's leadership and tireless efforts fundraising for NYRR youth programs epitomize the giving spirit of Team for Kids. It's thanks to him, and fundraisers like him, that we are able to reach thousands of kids every year with our life-changing programs."

Looking ahead, Swiss knows he has to change a few things in his routine if he wants to keep running. In his late fifties he started to notice injuries creeping in. He had a hip flexor strain in 2015. He also suffered three herniated discs, but he attributes that to computer use, not running. His doctor told him he shouldn't run anymore, but Swiss is having none of that. He found a rehab doctor, a former Israeli Army commando, who put him through some grueling sessions and told him to get out and keep running. He's experimented with the program detailed in *Run Less, Run Faster* and thinks that it may be the way for him now. "When I was young, even through my forties, I could run ten miles without hydrating. I never stretched, never cross-trained, and never took a day off," says Swiss. "Now, I take two days off, hydrate on every run, cross-train with cycling and weights, and only run thirty-five miles a week when I'm not in marathon training." He's experimented with his nutrition, and in 2016, after seeing the documentary *Forks over Knives*, he became a vegan. He still struggles with getting enough protein but is dedicated to figuring it out.

Swiss's goal for 2018 is to better his 2017 New York City Marathon time, and he is dedicated to that end. He's looking into getting a personal coach. He'll work with a nutritionist to lose fifteen more pounds, which would bring him down to his high school wrestling weight. As with his fundraising efforts, he is relentless. But he can also be quite emotional. When he received the award for top fundraiser at the 2017 TFK pre-marathon breakfast, he stood up in front of more two thousand people, which included his wife and kids, and broke down. When he finishes his marathons with TFK and comes into the post-marathon tent, he is greeted with cheers. His teammates know how much heart he has put into his effort. They also appreciate how he has taken on the mission and made it his personal goal to raise as much as he can for the kids.

Swiss applies his work ethic, honed at such a young age, toward getting in the necessary training for his marathons and also to managing his fundraising. He's also full of surprises. Two years ago, in the post-marathon tent, he stripped off his TFK singlet to reveal a gnarly tattoo on his upper right arm. Everyone who saw it was shocked. Mild-mannered, suit-and-tie Drew Swiss sporting a badass tattoo of a cobra with his name on it? There had to be a backstory: when he was fourteen and trying to fit in with the older, cooler street kids, a friend who had a tattoo took Swiss to get one of his own—and a Mohawk haircut to complete the look. "I regretted it the next day," he laughs. The Mohawk was reversible, but the tattoo remains.

His 2018 goals include running the United NYRR Half Marathon in March, which he completed in 2:12. His future dream is to someday run a marathon with his kids. That's not such a stretch, as his whole family runs. His wife, Amy, has run two marathons and the kids are now getting into road races. Through his dedication to fundraising and determined pursuit of his goals, he has been a role model not only to his family and friends but to countless underserved kids who are the beneficiaries of his tireless efforts. At sixty, Swiss has miles and miles to go before he calls it a day.

Kathrine Switzer

DOB: January 5, 1947

Residences: Wellington, New Zealand, and New Paltz, New York

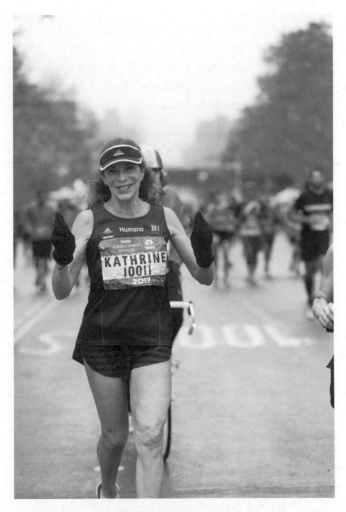

Kathrine Switzer

"The marathon woman."

Any runner who came on to the running scene in the seventies, especially women, should be familiar with Kathrine Switzer, one of the pioneers of women's running. The iconic photograph of Switzer being body blocked by Jock Semple, the unofficial race director of the Boston Marathon who tried to forcefully throw her out of his all-male race in 1967, hit the wire service and global newspapers, transforming her life overnight from college student to forceful activist who fought hard and relentless for the inclusion of women in events from the Boston Marathon to the Olympic Marathon.

Switzer was the first female to run with a bib, which set off Semple, a feisty Scotsman. He ignored Roberta Gibb, who in 1966 jumped on the course without a bib a few yards after the start. She ran the course, cheered and supported by the men and finished in 3:21:40, although her time was never recorded. Switzer registered for the race as K.V. Switzer and received a bib. On race-day morning she passed without notice through the corrals wearing a bulky sweatshirt and sweatpants on a cold, rainy morning. She was more than prepared to run the 26.2 miles having trained through the brutal winters at Syracuse University, running up to thirty-one miles just to be sure she could go the distance. She needed to prove she could do it not just for herself but for every female who was told she couldn't run a marathon.

Switzer waited five years to return to Boston in 1972, the year women were officially allowed to run the event. Nina Kuscsik won with Switzer finishing third. She upped her training and in 1974 won the New York City Marathon in 3:07:49. Switzer has been a fixture in women's sports for five decades and isn't slowing down. She went back to Boston in 2017 to run the fiftieth anniversary of her explosive debut and to launch her latest endeavor, 261 Fearless, a global supportive social running network that empowers women to connect and take control of their lives through the freedom gained by running. "Running is a social revolution now. Women are not just doing it to get into races or to lose a couple of pounds, they're doing it for fun, for self-esteem. It's transformative," she said. "We've come a light-year but we still have a long way to go." She is still running marathons today.

Kathrine Virginia Switzer was raised in Virginia, the only daughter and second child of a military father and guidance counselor mother. She was taught at an early age to be independent and make her own way into the world. In high school, when she wanted to try out for the cheerleading squad, her father responded, "Why do you want to cheer for others? You should be doing a sport where others cheer for you." This was in the early 1950s and sports for girls were very limited. She thought about field hockey but struggled with the skill set involved. Her father suggested she concentrate on becoming the fastest on the team and not to worry about handling the stick. With her "can-do" attitude, and running a mile a day, she became the fastest member of the team. No one could catch her as she sprinted down the field. At Lynchburg College in 1965, she kept up her running and joined the boys' track team, clocking a 5:58 mile while getting hooted and cat-called by the boys in the dorm that overlooked the track. In 1966 she transferred to Syracuse University to pursue her dream of becoming a sportswriter. She asked to be an unofficial member of the men's cross-country team and held her own in practice.

While at Syracuse she found a mentor in Arnie Briggs, a volunteer coach for the team. He took her under his wing and together they ran after practice to get in more miles. It wasn't unusual for them to run eight to ten miles a day. Briggs taught her everything he knew about running distance. At first she struggled to keep up but soon was matching him stride for stride. Briggs had run the Boston Marathon fifteen times and on their long runs he entertained her with stories of the fabled marathon, as well as coaching advice. Under his tutelage Switzer became a running machine.

As the legendary story goes, one day while out on a run and hearing Briggs tell his umpteenth story about Boston, Switzer snapped and said, "Damn it Arnie, let's quit talking about the Boston Marathon and run the damn thing!" He replied that no woman can run the Boston Marathon. Even Briggs thought the distance too long for women. When Switzer pointed out that Gibb had run it, he was still adamant, but softened a bit and said, "If any woman can do it, you can." The rest, as they say, is history. On Wednesday, April 19, Patriot's Day in Boston, Switzer radicalized the concept of women marathoners. The night before the marathon she called her father for moral support. The man who told her not to be a cheerleader but to do something where people cheered for her could not have imagined this day when crowds in Boston and then the world would be cheering for her.

After Semple tried to knock her out of the race, Switzer felt nauseous and unnerved. She thought she might even get arrested. This was more than the nineteen-year-old imagined would happen just because she wanted to run a marathon. As she writes in her memoir, *Marathon Woman*, "I knew if I quit, nobody would ever believe that women had the capability to run twenty-six-plus miles. If I quit, everybody would say it was a publicity stunt. If I quit, it would set women's sports back, way back, instead of forward. If I quit, I'd never run Boston. If I quit, Jock Semple and all those like him would win. My fear and humiliation turned to anger." The next day with her face and story plastered on global headlines, she was feted and in demand for her story. She was on *The Tonight Show Starring Johnny Carson* and *The Today Show with Gene Shalit*. But her mind was racing not on this one event but what she had unleashed. "I've stepped into a different life," she says.

After Switzer ran the 1972 Boston Marathon, she got involved with the emerging running scene in New York, becoming part of the original fabric of New York Road Runners. She also became a sportscaster and co-narrated the first Olympic Women's Marathon in Los Angeles in 1984 as thousands of women looking on in Los Angeles and around the world cheered and cried as Joan Benoit Samuelson won the first-ever gold medal in the event. Switzer was part of the small team of female runners who spent years lobbying the International Olympic Committee (IOC) for women's inclusion in the Olympic Marathon. She used her platform at Avon, where she was handpicked to be their first Director of Sports and Public Relations for Avon Running Events, to organize the first women's marathon in Atlanta in 1978. Under Switzer, Avon-sponsored running events ultimately expanded into 427 countries on three continents and twenty-seven countries on five continents. "This was entirely a 'Build It, and They Will Come' moment," laughs Switzer. The proof that women were running marathons became part of the supporting data Switzer brought the IOC, along with medical reports to dispel the myth that marathons were harmful to women. "This group of old men really thought that women would end up fainting or worse if we ran a marathon," recalls Switzer. "We actually had to have data to prove that a woman's uterus would not fall out."

After the hard fight for women's inclusion into the Olympics—which Switzer felt was the culmination of her career—Switzer concentrated on her sports commentary of other Olympic events, plus major world marathons. Her articles appeared in major publications and she wrote *Marathon Woman*, on her running life. She developed into a dynamic and effective speaker, convincing roomfuls of women that yes, they can run a marathon.

To get in shape for her historic 2017 Boston Marathon fifty years after her first one, she trained by running repeats around a cricket field in Wellington, New Zealand, where she spends half the year with her husband, Rodger Robinson. "If I finish breathless, I know I've had a good workout," describes Switzer. She swears by Yasso 800s (predicting your marathon time based on how long it takes to you to run 800 meters). "I think more than anything they got me in top shape for the marathon and for running a great time." Gone are the days when she and her running buddies ran ten marathons a year. She runs by time now, not mileage. She's also become an advocate of core workouts and keeps a set of dumbbells at each house. Her biggest struggle is getting enough sleep. With all her projects and initiatives and "constant dirty house," she's lucky if she manages five hours a night. Seven hours is like a mini-vacation.

When asked about the changes she's seen in women's running since 1967, she doesn't hesitate to give a long and empowering response. "In the last fifty years I've seen the emergence of women taking control of their lives through running in ways they never could before. I can't tell you what it means to me to see millions of women running and for reasons other than losing weight. They feel empowered and makes them feel they can achieve anything in life," says Switzer. "It's turned into a social revolution and women are feeling fearless." She continues: "I'm pleased to see the emergence of women's running in cultures beyond the United States such as Africa and Malaysia, where women are second-class citizens at best. She points to the world-class Kenyan women marathoners like Tegla Loroupe and Edna Kiplagat who have invested their prize money into education for children and women. Loroupe, the first African woman to win a major marathon, the 1994 New York City Marathon, founded the Tegla Loroupe Peace Foundation, an international humanitarian charity to promote peacebuilding, livelihoods, and resilience of poor people affected by and vulnerable to conflicts and civil strife. Edna Kiplagat, winner of the Los Angeles (2010), New York (2010), London (2014), and Boston (2017) Marathons started the Edna Kiplagat Foundation to raise awareness of breast cancer. This would never have happened without the opportunities for these women to run in marathons and then inspire other women from other countries to train and enter marathons. "The women's marathon movement has changed the landscape of the world," adds Switzer.

Back home, Switzer saw the emergence of groups such as Black Girls Run, started in 2009 as a grassroots organization that encourages and inspires African-American women to live a healthy lifestyle. The seeds for Switzer's 261 Fearless, named for her Boston bib number, began in 2012 when Switzer started to notice emails and letters from women all over the world thanking her for inspiring them to take up running. Some started out, "Dear Kathrine, I too have felt unwelcomed or told I couldn't do something like run. Thank you for being fearless and now I am too." The letters all stemmed from a new generation of women who saw the photos of Switzer getting knocked by Semple in 1967. Others letters read, "People make fun of me because I am a girl but I am running my first marathon because of you." These letters were coming from women in countries that have historically abused women or kept them under control with no laws to protect them.

Eventually she was asked to spearhead the emerging movement. "I wasn't looking to ignite another revolution but saw the need," explains Switzer. "I agreed to kick it off but couldn't run the daily operations. It was the moral thing to do. Like a baby, I needed to nurture it and then watch it grow."

The official kickoff for 261 Fearless was targeted for Switzer's 2017 Boston Marathon event. The BAA helped out by offering a number of the coveted bibs as a fundraiser for the non-profit. "I think this was their moment to really apologize to me for what happened in 1967," laughs Switzer. On that one day, the group raised more than $800,000. The organization is now in thirteen countries with a website in different languages to reach out to all women.

Switzer is taking her aging in stride and not letting it slow her down. She's still out there running marathons (London 2018) and is booked globally for speaking engagements about her new endeavor and her life. She has accepted aging gracefully, crepey skin and all. "I'm so far removed from what my body looks like," she laughs. "I can still run marathons and work around the clock so women globally can feel fearless. Who cares about pasty, crepey skin?" She's ready to pass the torch to these women who will take the movement forward. "I've never felt so exited about something as I do now at seventy-one years old," says

Switzer. "I've always believed that putting one foot in front of the other and following your dream can lead to change."

Reflecting on her life, she's most proud of showing women that through running they can change their lives for the better. Switzer has dedicated fifty-two years of her life to making a difference for women and is not about to stop. She would like to have a cleaner house and more sleep but that will come.

Kathryn Waldron

DOB: March 13, 1959

Residence: Green Bay, Wisconsin

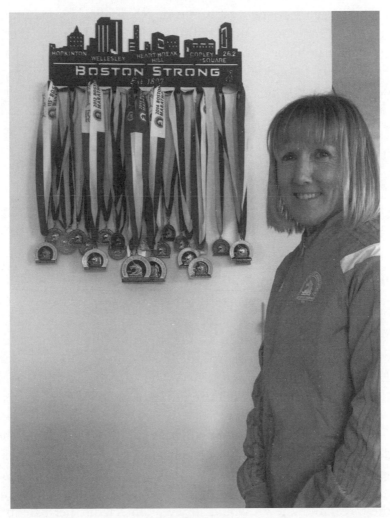

Kathy Waldron

"Embrace life and all it has to offer."

Kathy Waldron is a member of the exclusive Boston Marathon Quarter Century Club, having run twenty-five straight Boston Marathons as of the 2016 Boston Marathon. The Boston Athletic Association has just seventy-six streakers as of 2017 and Waldron is only one of six females on the list. To add to her celebration that day, Waldron not only accomplished the twenty-five-year mark, it was also her one-hundredth marathon. Waldron, who has two adult children and two grandkids, had a lot to celebrate that day.

Waldron grew up on a farm outside Reedsville, Wisconsin, which had a population of fewer than 2,500 people when she was living there. She was sixth in line of twelve kids. She credits growing up on a farm were her ability to buckle down and stay the course for the long haul. "We all had chores from the time we could walk," laughs Waldron. "We had to pitch in and make the farm work as it was our livelihood. We were really poor." With twelve kids, she wasn't in need of playmates. They never had toys, relying on boxes and other items that they made into toys. I asked what it was like to be one of twelve, and she has nothing but praise for her siblings, stating they are her best friends. "We were very close. We had to be as there were usually three in a bed most years. Only the oldest brother had his own room, which was really just a big closet, but he felt like he had a suite."

On weekends while other kids were playing sports or enjoying time off from school, Waldron and her siblings worked even longer hours. Plus, "There are no summer vacations for farmers." School was tough. She was picked on and tormented for being poor, for her hand-me-down clothes and shy manner. Taking the school bus was torture. The kids smashed her lunch box, made fun of her clothes, and were relentless in their bullying and teasing. On days when she missed the school bus and had to be driven to school in an old Ford station wagon, it was even worse.

Looking back now from the perspective of a tough marathoner, single parent, and now a grandmother, she wouldn't change it for anything. "My upbringing is what prepared me for life. When I divorced and had to raise two kids on my own with no money, I just picked up the pieces and knew I would survive." She credits her parents with instilling in her a strong work ethic and figuring things out for herself. Her father dropped out of school after eighth grade to tend full time to the farm. But he spent any free time at the library, reading books on all topics. He was a voracious reader and learner. At the time of his death he was learning Spanish. Her mother, a nurse, worked the night shift at a hospital.

In seventh grade, the class had to do a running drill and she beat everyone, even the boys. A girl in her class was impressed with her speed and told her she should go out for track. "It was the first time a class-mate said something nice to me so I took notice," she recalls. Waldron became a middle-distance running standout in high school. Specializing in the 880-yard and mile runs, she qualified for state and in 1975, won the one-mile run with a time of 5:24. The school didn't have a girl's cross country team but the boy's coach used her as a rabbit for the boys to chase.

Her dad took notice of her running ability and told her about the Boston Marathon, saying that she should run it some day. He bragged to everyone about how fast his daughter was. When she was nineteen, he did some research in the library about females running a marathon and came across an article of Kathrine Switzer at the 1967 Boston Marathon. He made a copy of the article and gave it to her daughter with a note saying that some day she would run the Boston Marathon. "I still have that note," says Waldron.

She credits her father with most of her strength and gumption in life and reflects on him often during our interview: "Pa was a brave and clever man. When he took the old station wagon out he always parked it on a hill so he could 'pop the clutch' and get it started just in case. When we were all piled in the car and started getting too restless and fighting with each other, Pa would stop the car—no matter the weather or where we were—and kick us out of the car and drive one mile ahead. By the time we ran our mile back to the car, we were laughing so hard we could hardly breathe! Pa was a smart man! Many of my family members are runners today and I attribute this at least partially to his unorthodox training technique!"

Graduating high school in 1977, Waldron went to school to be-come a ward clerk at a hospital. She continued running, entering local 5Ks and 10Ks. She married in 1979 and had two kids. In 1987, she attempted to run a marathon, putting in one-hundred-mile weeks. She had to get up at 3:00 a.m. to get in her runs so she could be back in time to get the kids to school. By the time she was tapering for the marathon, she was physically and mentally exhausted. On race day, she dropped out at mile 20. "I felt broken," says Waldron. Looking back she knows she overtrained but had no clue how to train for a marathon at the time. She simply thought, *more miles are better.* The woman who won put in half the training miles she did. It took her four years and a divorce in 1989 to start thinking of another marathon. And when she made her comeback, it was a big one.

Remembering the stories her father told her about the Boston Marathon, she decided to run it in 1992. She trained smarter by cutting back on the weekly mileage. Her eight-year-old daughter Sarah accompanied her on her bike during training runs. When she qualified for Boston at the Fox Cities Marathon in 1991 her kids were at the finish line and screamed, "We're going to Boston!" When she told her father he said he would run it with her, but as a bandit, or an unofficial runner. An avid runner himself and a strong proponent of an active lifestyle, he wanted to share the day with her. They hung out in the Athlete's Village and then found each other at the finish. It was one of the highlights in her life to run that marathon. "I lived on that joy for a whole year," says Waldron. A year later, her father died from prostate cancer. As a tribute to him, he was buried with her Boston Marathon medal. Her mother died the following year. "I feel them on my shoulders every year that I run Boston," says Waldron. "I know they are with me."

She started running other marathons, those she could get to by driving, even if it meant sleeping in her car. She stopped at truck stops, which she found safer than motels rooms. "It's so quite and peaceful, the best way to travel," says Waldron. Now a single parent, Waldron worked in the medical field to make ends meet. In 2005 she learned how to drive an eighteen-wheeler and took a job driving across the country.

In 2010 she ran eight marathons—three in a span of six weeks— placing first in her age division at five of them. She finished the year by driving to the Baton Rouge Marathon, where she placed first in her age division in 3:28:58 at age fifty-one. In one of the few races in which she did not win her age group she was outpaced by Joan Benoit Samuelson, Olympic Gold Medalist and two-time winner of the Boston Marathon. Waldron placed a respectable second, following Samuelson. Afterward, Waldron commented, "It's a great accomplishment to place second to Joanie."

Every year since 1992 she returned to Boston. It wasn't until she ran her nineteenth Boston Marathon that she realized she could be a serious contender for the Quarter Century Club. She's had three close calls that almost ended her streak. One year she was having foot pain before the race so extreme she could barely walk. She managed to get through the marathon and then had it taken care of. During the 2011 Boston Marathon registration, she didn't have a computer and asked her son to enter her. He did, but then a computer glitch wiped out all her data entry. Frantic, she put in a call to someone who could help and her name reappeared on the entry registration.

In 2014, she slipped on a patch of ice in her driveway and suffered a bone bruise on her right knee and couldn't run for six weeks right before the marathon. She drove to Boston, ran the first half at a slow pace, and then shuffled through the second half, finishing in 4:54, her worst time ever (her best time was 3:01 in 1998 at age thirty-nine). "That was so painful, but I cannot tell you how thankful I was to still participate," Waldron says.

For her twenty-fifth Boston Marathon, her brother Bill, his wife Julie, her sister Nettie, Nettie's husband Mark, and her daughter Sarah and three-year-old grandson McCoy all came to see her run. As a special surprise, her brother Jim flew in the morning of the marathon and surprised her at the finish. "Having my family there was one of the best moments of very special weekend," exclaims Waldron. Her twenty-seventh Boston Marathon was April 2018, which had one of the worst weather conditions in years. Waldron recalls the day: "Of all twenty-seven Boston runs this was by far the most brutal. But I can't tell you how thankful I am to have kept my streak alive! It was a slow run with a finish time of 4:12, due to age and very strong headwinds but I wouldn't have missed it for the world!"

As Waldron ages, she follows a simple philosophy, not much different than how she has always treated her running. She runs by herself and has never joined a running club or hired a coach. She doesn't wear a watch. "All those beeps would drive me crazy," she laughs. She stays off pavement as much as she can, preferring to run on the soft pine needles in a park by her house.

"As long as I live, I hope I can always keep doing it," says Waldron with passion. "I take every step as it comes." The family farm is now owned by a sister and brother-in-law. All the siblings come back to the farm for holidays. "We love getting together at the farm with our own kids and spouses for Thanksgiving and other holidays," she exclaims. "We still build big bonfires and tell stories of when we were kids." She feels so lucky to have her siblings in her life and in her running. One of her brothers wants to run his first marathon with Waldron and she is tickled silly to help him. Her grandson also talks about running his first marathon with her one day.

Toward the close of our interview, Waldron takes a pause—she talks as fast as she runs—and reflects on her running life. The years of middle school bullying and then an unhappy marriage has left her scared and she admits to being a loner. "Running is a sport that is great for loners because you don't need a team. I can do my own thing," she explains. "But when I go to the same races year in and year out I see familiar faces and we reconnect over our love for running. It has opened up a whole new world for me. It's just a neat, neat sport."

On the back of every race bib, Waldron writes a scripture verse that was passed down to her from her dad at that very first Boston Marathon in 1992. It's a passage from the prophet Habakkuk, and found in the Hebrew Bible: "The Sovereign Lord is my strength; he makes my feet like the feet of a deer; he enables me to tread on the heights" (Habakkuk 3:19). The passage is decidedly apropos for Waldron. She has the swift feet of a deer and her passion for running has brought her to heights in her life she never dreamed. From being bullied and shy, she now has many running friends she looks forward to seeing at races and has her entire family cheering for her and helping with race entries and fees if needed. Her marathon photos show a petite, smiling, happy woman with thumbs up embracing life and all it has to offer.

Ed Whitlock

DOB: March 6, 1931
Died: March 13, 2017

Residence: Milton, Ontario

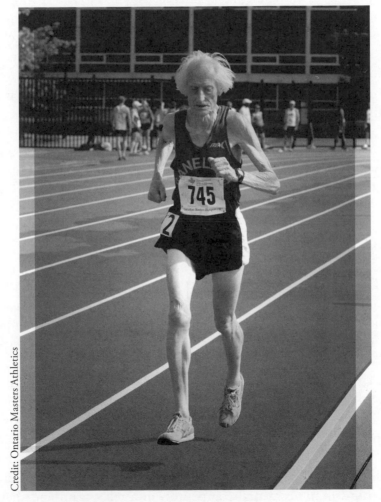

Ed Whitlock

The Accidental Marathoner Turned World-Record Holder.
Soft-spoken, lean, and handsome in a bygone Hollywood-leading-man kind of way, Whitlock is humble about his world records, shy, very polite, and always the gentleman. He has a bit of a dry wit as well. The morning of our interview, it's the day after Halloween, and Whitlock reveals something to me no other journalist knows: he is eating the leftover Halloween candy. Yes, Ed Whitlock has a sweet tooth. He is human after all. He got into marathons accidentally when his then fifteen-year-old son wanted to run one. "I was just an old miler, never a marathoner," he says. "But I thought he might get hurt so I wanted to run it with him." Forty years later, Whitlock set an age-division world record, running a 3:56:34 at the Scotiabank Toronto Waterfront Marathon in October 9, 2016, at eighty-five.

To understand this running outlier, who holds more world records than he can keep track of and defies convention, is to go back to his roots growing up in England. He ran track and cross-country while attending London University where he majored in mining. His best time for the miler was 4:31 when he was seventeen and was a champion three-miler with a time of 14:54. He knew he had talent, but upon graduation he moved to Canada. "At that time, England was only mining coal, which I had no interest in doing, so I immigrated to Canada to mine metal," recalls Whitlock. "No one ran in northern Ontario" he says. "I wasn't ambitious enough to run on my own and missed the camaraderie of a team. This was 1952, before anyone heard of a running boom."

Twenty years later, married with two young boys, he got back into the sport in a backward sort of way. It was sports day at his son's school and his wife volunteered to help out. When she learned they were short a running coach for one of the events, she volunteered Whitlock for the job. Once at the track, he ran a few laps to see if he still had it and surprised himself. His level of fitness was above average due to his gardening, lots of walking, refereeing of his boys' soccer games, and lots of shoveling snow. Gradually, he added more running and enjoyed showing up at the track and running with the teenagers. After they got to know Whitlock, they asked him to be on a relay team with them as they were short a body. After twenty years for quitting the sport, Whitlock found himself an accidental competitor on a relay team and they did quite well. "Slowly, the bug to run full time and get competitive was nipping at me," said Whitlock.

This was in 1972 and the first running boom and masters movement was just beginning to take hold in the United States, but not Canada. "Older runners and cyclists were consider weird," says Whitlock. "It was still a sport for kids, not adults." The World Amateur Veterans Association (WAVA) was just forming and held the first world championships in 1975 in Toronto. Whitlock was there. In 2001 the name changed to the World Masters Association (WMA), and he became part of the Canadian executive management team. He started running and competing regularly in the 800- and 1500-meter events. "Ironically, I ran faster times as a master than I ever did as a kid," says Whitlock.

He owes his marathon career to his son Clive who at age fifteen wanted to tackle a marathon. Whitlock was concerned about his young age so he decided to accompany him. "I didn't seriously train for this," he says. "I knew an 800-meter runner had no business running a marathon. My longest run was fifteen miles." The marathon was in March and bitter cold. There were four hundred participants and no water stops. Clive hit the wall at mile 22 but pushed forward. Whitlock would have been happy to quit. They finished in 3:09.

Three months later they did another one and finished in 2:56. The following year, 1977, they won the father-son team competition at the Ottawa Marathon, finishing in 2:52. Clive was seventeen and Ed was forty-six. Clive decided to quit running after that but his older brother Neil decided he wanted to run a marathon with dad. They ran the Ottawa Marathon the following year in 2:48. Neil still runs competitively.

Never having intended to run one marathon, in the course of two years, Whitlock ran four, three of them under three hours. In 1979, Whitlock decided to test himself and put in one-hundred-mile weeks building up to the Montreal Marathon. He finished in 2:33, placing second, at age forty-eight. Two months later he ran a 2:31 at Ottawa, his personal best. But even after proving his prowess in the marathon, he still considered himself a track guy. The same year he ran his marathon PR he won the 1500 meters at the WAVA world championships. Looking at his gold medal, he commented: "Professionally speaking I don't think there was much gold in that medal. It wouldn't have passed the bite test."

During those years Whitlock was working full-time, raising a family, and putting in the training. He would go out for a run at 10:00 p.m. in the dark and cold to get his miles in. "There was no money in it for me so I guess I really did enjoy it," he recalls. He took on marathon training full-time after retirement, but didn't add anything new to his regime of running a three-mile loop around a cemetery near his home. He doesn't do speed work, no hill repeats, doesn't cross-train, and never stretches. Aches and pains? He just waits until they go away. "I don't dislike training, but I don't look forward to it either," he says. "I get nervous and feel awful before an important race and then when it is over I feel euphoric, especially if I have done well. I don't want to embarrass myself."

I doubt there has ever been a time that Whitlock embarrassed himself at a race. At sixty-nine, he became the oldest person to break three hours for the marathon. He got a compliment from Bill Rodgers on that occasion. He tried to do it again at age seventy but was injured and missed the three-hour mark by twenty-three seconds. His 2:54 marathon at age seventy-three is considered one of the greatest age-group performances of all time and is the one he is most proud of, describing it a magical day when everything came together. A year later he ran a 2:58 marathon. Whitlock never disappoints. He credits his ability with good genes. "It all comes down to good genes and I was blessed," he says. "That and perseverance."

He doesn't have rituals, has never taken an ice bath and doesn't run at a set time every day. "It depends on how I feel on any given day," says Whitlock. "I don't make a fetish about it." He doesn't give out advice. His next goal is to just keep running as long as he can. He gets philosophical when asked about being eighty-five: "I don't quite buy into the saying that age is just a number. I'm old. I have arthritis. But I really don't fixate on it. I'm aging as well as I can and get the same aches and pains as every other eighty-five-year-old. Maybe my running has helped me stay in shape, maybe not." He doesn't go to doctors. The last one he saw was ten years ago for a knee injury, which wasn't running related. He had an MRI taken and the doctor told him he would never run again.

When asked what has changed for him since he started setting world records, he says that now race directors put him up for free. "I'm not a hero or a celebrity," he says with a bit of frustration. "Even though the world has broadcast my life, I like to think I am a very simple man. All this attention is a bit embarrassing." He has also noticed that the medals are getting larger, and it seems that everyone gets one. He keeps most of his medals in a drawer with the exception of a small, silver one he won while at university. It's made from real silver.

Like most competitive runners, he dissects every race and analyzes how he could have done better, whether he set a record or not. At his last world-record race in Toronto, he felt he could have run five minutes faster if it weren't for the windy conditions and if he had used better pacing judgment. He prefers looped, flat, fast courses, which is why he says he has never run the Boston or New York Marathons.

Along with being the most famous outlier in road racing, Whitlock just enjoys running and being part of the running community. "Runners are universally good people with great spirits and very supportive," he says. "I enjoy their company."

His death in March of 2017 was a shock to most but some close to him knew about his cancer. Sports writer Scott Douglas posted a note about Whitlock in *Runner's World* online: "Ed Whitlock, the Canadian runner who rewrote the record books and forever altered conceptions of human endurance performance in older age, died on Monday in Toronto, not far from his home in Milton, Ontario. Whitlock was 86." Whitlock was admired by all and was also a bit of an enigma to doctors at the Mayo Clinic who declared him "as close as you can get to minimal aging in a human being." He was also humble and couldn't understand why people saw him as an inspiration. "I just run" is how he responded to reporters' questions about his speed and endurance at his age. Whitlock will live on in the history books and records. And despite his unwillingness to see himself as an inspiration and role model, he will be one forever.

Motivating Factors

Webster's Dictionary defines the word motivation as "the reason or reasons one has for acting or behaving in a particular way; the general desire or willingness of someone to do something; and the act or process of giving someone a reason for doing something."

In his 1968 Theory of Goal Setting, Dr. Edwin Locke, a University of Maryland professor and pioneering researcher on goal setting and motivation, stated:

> Research supports predictions that the most effective performance seems to result when goals are specific and challenging, when they are used to evaluate performance and linked to feedback on results, and create commitment and acceptance. Deadlines improve the effectiveness of goals. A learning goal orientation leads to higher performance than a performance goal orientation, and group goal-setting is as important as individual goal-setting.

For runners, motivation comes from anywhere and everywhere—whether it be a place deep in our hearts, a rebellion against rules, or keeping a streak alive. If you are a female of a certain age, say before Title IX passed, motivation came from being told you couldn't do something, like run. Pioneers such as Kathrine Switzer, Nina Kuscsik, and Julia Chase stood up against the male-dominated rules and boycotted for equality. Don't tell them and the hundreds like them who hid their running at night or jumped into the Boston Marathon from the bushes that they can't run. Their motivation led to the inclusion of women in the Boston Marathon in 1972, won by Nina Kuscsik, and to Joan Benoit Samuelson becoming the first Olympic winner of the women's marathon in 1984. Those voices, and more that joined the chorus in the 1960s and 1970s, started the ball rolling for females to lace up their shoes and hit the road. According to USATF statistics, today 57 percent of all race entries from the 5K to the marathon are female.

Julia Chase

DOB: August 24, 1942

Residence: New London, Connecticut

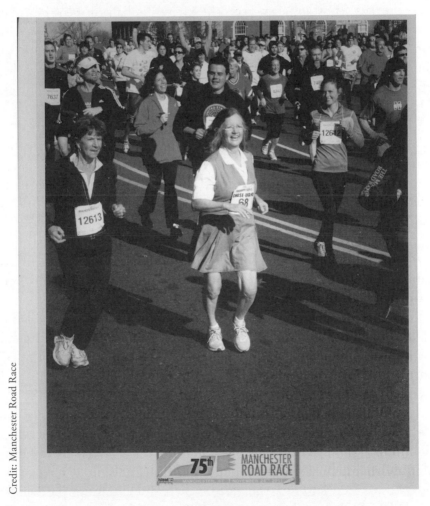

Julia Chase

"Be defiant."

Julia Chase grew up running through the woods and along the shores of Long Island Sound near her Groton, Connecticut, home. In Amby Burfoot's book *First Ladies of Running*, he profiles Chase: "As a teenager she spent most of her time outdoors with her four brothers. As the middle child in a family of all boys, Julia learned quickly to pick up a variety of sports with a skill that rivaled most boys her age." She ran effortlessly and fast. At fourteen, she learned that one of her neighbors was the legendary marathoner John J. Kelley. When she learned he had won the 1957 Boston Marathon, she knew she had to meet him. She started running along the same streets and routes in hopes of meeting him and one day she got her opportunity and introduced herself. Being the friendly and enthusiastic guy he was, he stopped to talk with her. They talked about running and he encouraged her to race. Kelley, like Chase, was also defiant and thought she should be able to do whatever she wanted with her running.

Kelley and his running buddy George Terry took her under their wing and taught her about running. They traveled to track meets throughout New England where she ran the 800 meters, one of the few distances women were allowed to run according to AAU rules at the time. Recognizing her talent, they entered her into the 1960 US Olympic 800 meters Track Trials. This was the first time since 1928 that women were allowed to run the 800 meters, so the excitement and participation level were high. Terry accompanied her to Abilene, Texas, for the Trials.

This was her only second 800-meter race and she was a bit out of her league among the seasoned and talented runners such as the legendary Wilma Rudolph. Despite her dedication and enthusiasm, she placed fifth. She and Terry continued to travel to track meets where she dominated in local 400- and 800-meter races.

Her biggest event yet was going to be the 1960 Thanksgiving Day Manchester Road Race, an all-male five-mile race in Manchester, Connecticut. The morning of the race, Kelley and Terry drove her to Manchester where Kelley was a popular and many-times winner of the race. To all their surprise, she was blocked from running the race by AAU officials. Women belonged only on the track and up to 800 meters, she was told. Disappointed, she didn't challenge the officials. Instead, she watched her friends run the race and then went home. She was soothed somewhat by their comments that she could have easily beaten half the field. She went back to Smith College and plotted her revenge.

The following year, 1961, she went back and this time was not going to be dismissed. But once again, the race directors refused her entry to their race. She was polite but firmly let them know she was running their race anyway. She edged into the crowd and found two other women who were also charged up to run. One was Chris McKenzie, a well-known British middle-distance runner and the other was Dianne Lechausse, a dancer. As much as the race director and his cronies tried to block them from running, they kept weaving around them and eventually settled into the race. Flying by the men in her Smith College gym shorts, spectators on the course cheered for her, which encouraged her to run faster.

Julia recalls that day: "Six weeks before the race, the papers found out that my coach George Terry had again sent in my application to run Manchester and had once again been turned down. This time we decided to defy the AAU rules and announced that I intended to run anyway. Intense press coverage started. After thirty years of being banned from running more than the sprint distances, American women were frustrated with the arbitrary limits imposed by the 'Big Boys of the AAU.' The roads were public property—mine as much as my brother's. My mother's family were Quaker and active in suffrage. And only five years before my Manchester Race, Rosa Parks had demonstrated the effectiveness of civil disobedience. So I would run.

"What I didn't realize was how intense this stand-off would become. Somehow it resonated with people: I was pretty and young; I wasn't threatening anyone, so why shouldn't I be allowed to run? The story spread from local papers to the *New York Times*, and then worldwide on AP and Reuters. Soon I was receiving requests from a Finnish nudist to send an outline of my bare feet (I complied). A South-African woman wrote to encourage me, saying her aunt used to run to market weekly in the 1930s. And lonely GIs from Japan and children from the Midwest wrote to encourage me to run. I was being interviewed daily and soon *Life* magazine and *Sports Illustrated* sent reporters who followed me to class at Smith. I was a media freak and felt intensely alone—but it was wrong that I couldn't run, and I stuck to my guns. Boxes and boxes of letters appeared at my dorm room. And in the background was the AAU, threatening that I would be banned from all amateur sports if I ran.

"On race day, I was scared and excited. Scared because I didn't know if I was going to be handcuffed or physically pushed off the road, and excited because it was finally showtime. Thousands of spectators and swarms of TV and press reporters were there . . . and then the surprise, two other women had shown up. Chris McKenzie, an English middle-distance runner, and Diane Lechausse, a ballet dancer who was a senior at Manchester High School, also decided to run. The officials tried to stop us but only succeeded in delaying our start as we ducked out of their grasp. The first man I passed warmly said "Way to go, girl." At the finish, the noise was thunderous, almost scary, and the press was spilling into the road, and I couldn't see the finish line.

"Afterward, I did cartwheels in my bare feet and George Terry carried me around piggy-back. We'd done it. After two months the AAU came back with a compromise: if I promised to never embarrass them on the roads again, they would not suspend me . . . and more importantly, they agreed to begin sanctioning women's cross-country running. After thirty years the US had caught up to Europe."

Chase finished the 4.7-mile course in 33:40, a 7:10 pace. She was jubilant and was featured in the *New York Times* the next day.

Chase continued running and tried out for the 1964 US Olympic Trials 800 meter but failed to make the team. She graduated from Smith and went on to earn her PhD in zoology, teaching at Barnard College in Manhattan and Rutgers College in New Jersey. In 1981 she returned to Manchester, which was by then open to all runners. In 2011, the fiftieth anniversary of her first Manchester race, she returned to fanfare and media coverage. Running in the same Smith College gym shorts, she crossed the line in 51:32.

Julia Chase may not be a household name such as legendary female runners Nina Kuscsik and Kathrine Switzer, but she ranks up there with her courage, determination and steely resolve not to take no for an answer. And she did it years before any other female ran a road race. She still runs on the beaches near her New London home and tends to her garden. A retired psychiatrist, she is writing her memoirs and plays tennis with her husband.

Keep the Streak at All Costs

A strong motivator for runners is keeping a streak alive. Streaks can be defined as running every day or entering a certain race every year. Streak Runners International and United States Streak Association track runners who run at least one mile a day. According to a January 30, 2017, article in the *Washington Post*, the longest running streak in history by England's seventy-eight-year-old Ron Hill, a former Olympian, ended at 19,032 days. Starting on December 21, 1964, Hill ran at least a mile a day. That's fifty-two years and thirty-nine days. He ended the streak due to heart issues. That opens the path for Jon Sutherland, sixty-six, of West Hills, California, to overtake Hill's record. Sutherland now possesses the longest active streak in the world: 17,417 days, or forty-seven and a half years. Marathons have their streakers as well. Ben Beach, sixty-seven, ran his fiftieth consecutive Boston Marathon in 2017, the longest marathon streak recorded.

Brian Salzberg

DOB: September 4, 1942

Residence: Philadelphia, Pennsylvania

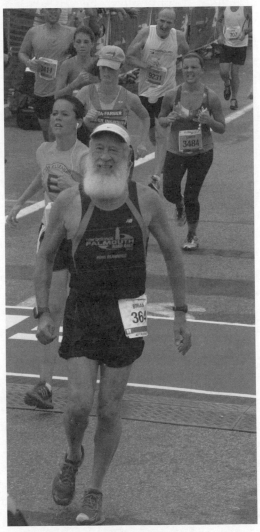

Brian Salzberg

"Last man standing?"

Brian Salzberg shares the record for the most consecutive Falmouth Road Races—forty-five—with a group of friends dubbed "the Falmouth Five." Salzberg, a professor of neuroscience and physiology at the Perelman School of Medicine at the University of Pennsylvania, went for his first run, a mere one mile, in Cambridge, Massachusetts while studying for his PhD at Harvard. He was inspired by Amby Burfoot's 1968 Boston Marathon win. Five years later in 1973 while a postdoc at Yale Medical School in physiology, he was working at the Marine Biological Laboratory in Woods Hole, Massachusetts, when he heard about a new race, the inaugural Falmouth Road Race. According to the Falmouth race website, the first Falmouth Road Race was held on a Wednesday afternoon to celebrate race founder Tommy Leonard's fortieth birthday and raise funds for the Falmouth High School girls' track team. Leonard designed the course to be seven miles—the distance from the Captain Kidd Restaurant in Woods Hole to the Brothers Four Pub, Tommy's workplace, in Falmouth Heights—and he spread information about what would become the "little race that could" by word of mouth—mainly his own. Ninety-three runners showed up for the race, which was billed as a marathon despite the fact that it was seven miles and quickly got the nickname, the "bar to bar" run.

Salzberg can recall his first Falmouth race like it was yesterday: "Best weather ever for a race: rain, wind, and temperatures in the mid-fifties plus a spectacularly beautiful course. There were no water stations, traffic cones, mile markers, or directional arrows. At the end of the race, wet and chilled runners crowded into The Brothers Four and partied until midnight. I can see so clearly in my mind Old Johnny Kelley—who was I think sixty-five then—spiffed up in a Hawaiian shirt jitterbugging with his wife." It was his first race, and Salzberg was hooked. Photos of Salzberg through the years on the Falmouth Road Race website show him aging gracefully. His Forrest Gump-esque beard gets longer and grayer with each year but the smile remains the same. He and four others hold the distinction of being the Falmouth Five, the only ones to have run all the Falmouth road races. Salzberg is the youngest, so he expects to be the last man standing.

Six weeks after running his first race he ran the 1973 New York City Marathon on September 30, which was four laps through Central Park. He thought he would BQ but the heat and the hills, plus poor pacing and a lack of training, did him in. So he found another marathon three weeks later, and BQed in his second attempt, running Boston in 1974. In his first year of running he completed six marathons. And he went back to Falmouth in 1974.

His streak has not been easy to keep alive. In 2003, he almost didn't make it to Falmouth. He underwent brain surgery for a nonmalignant tumor on his right cerebellum. After recovery he got clearance from his doctors to run the race. In 2008 badly sprained ligaments in his foot almost derailed the streak but determined to keep it alive, he completed the course on crutches. "That was my toughest race by far," he says. And his slowest, finishing in one hour and forty-nine minutes. He still has the crutches and the crutch course record.

But his biggest challenge to the streak came in 2010 when the tumor that was removed in 2003 came back. He underwent brain surgery in June, two months before the race, and returned to running two weeks later, but something wasn't right. He went back to the hospital and another operation was performed on the same site. "I think they held my skull together with chewing gum," laughs Salzberg. This time the doctors told him no running for six weeks. With the race in five weeks, Salzberg's biggest worry was how to keep the streak alive. His doctors reluctantly agreed to let him walk the course, wearing a heart monitor, which he did in one hour and forty-five minutes. The steak was alive and well. And to make sure the tumor never returns, he monitors the site by getting an annual MRI.

In his fifty years of running Salzberg has completed twenty-one marathons with a PR of two hours and forty-nine minutes at Boston in 1978. When asked what he is most proud of he claims running six marathons over a fifteen year period, from age thirty-five until age fifty, all under three hours, with a 2:58 at age fifty. And of course there is a story to go along with the last one. When he turned fifty, his buddies challenged him to run a marathon under three hours and they gave him a year to do it. Salzberg did it in his first attempt, running two hours and fifty-eight minutes and collecting $300.

Every August, he makes the six and a half hour drive from Philadelphia to Falmouth to continue the streak and see his friends. "Choosing to not run isn't an option," he says. "This is an unbreakable vow." In 2017 he completed his forty-fifth Falmouth Road Race. He is keeping his health and one day plans to be the Falmouth One.

Jonathan Mendes

DOB: November 3, 1920

Residence: Manhattan, New York

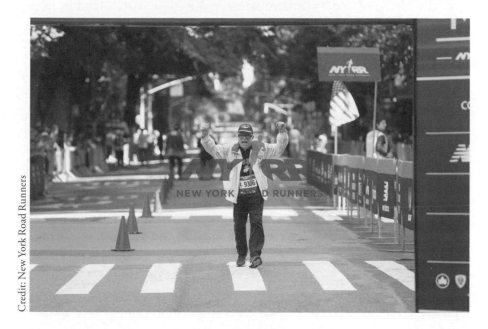

Jonathan Mendes

"We all need goals: twenty-six at ninety-six."

When Jonathan Mendes, a retired colonel in the United States Marine Corps who flew bomber missions in World War II and the Korean War, turned ninety-six, he decided to run the New York City Marathon, his sixteenth marathon overall and twelfth New York City Marathon. "You have to have goals in life," he explained when asked why he was running. "Without a goal, why get out of bed? It's no disgrace to fail, only not to try."

This isn't the first time Mendes has challenged himself with a big (some would say impossible) goal. In 2005 at age eighty-five, he was the oldest finisher at the New York City Marathon. In 2011 at age ninety-one he was the oldest finisher at the Marine Corps Marathon. At ninety-six, he was again the oldest finisher at New York, crossing the finish line in eleven hours and twenty minutes. He pretty much walked the 26.2 miles escorted by two guides. One was his personal trainer and the other a volunteer from Achilles International, which matches guides with disabled and older runners. They had a blast with Mendes, who entertained them along the route. Upon finishing he did his favorite post-marathon ritual while still in the recovery tent, propped up on a bed. When asked if he wanted some water or perhaps hot chocolate, he requested a scotch. Black Label if they had it.

When I called Mendes at his Manhattan home that overlooks Central Park, he answered the phone with a vibrant tone: "Jon Mendes here. What can I do for you?" I had interviewed Mendes a few years ago for a profile in *Runner's World* and we discovered that he was in the same Dartmouth class of 1942 as my father, creating an instant bond. Upon graduation, Mendes entered the war, becoming a US Marine bomber pilot. He flew more than one hundred missions in the Pacific and then flew jet fighter attack planes during the Korean War, earning a Distinguished Flying Cross for leading twenty-four attack aircraft in the bombing of a North Korean airfield. His flight jacket from his Korean missions is in the USMC National Museum in Virginia. He trained John Glenn and Ted Williams to become pilots. "We all saw the drive and determination in Glenn," he recalls. "He had all the right stuff and beyond for sure and was one heck of a nice guy."

After the war he entered Harvard Business School and became a successful investment banker. He and his wife raised a son and a daughter before she passed away after thirty-three years of marriage. A lifelong smoker, Mendes didn't engage in any physical activity beyond his intramural skiing days at Dartmouth. In 1966, feeling sluggish, his doctor warned him to quit his two-pack-a-day smoking habit and start exercising. He quit cold turkey and started running laps around the Central Park reservoir. At forty-six, he became a runner. He joined New York Road Runners and found a group of neighbors who were runners. They formed a club, the 72nd Street Marathoning and Pasta Club, and started running marathons. They also gave back to their beloved Central Park by planting trees and cleaning and restoring water fountains.

At ninety-seven, Mendes says he's done with marathons but has set a new goal: to inspire others of all ages to live a fit and healthy life. "Good health is not an accident," he says. "It is something you must strive for every day of your life." He should know. His weight, 160, is close to what he weighed in his college days. He still walks forty minutes in the morning through Central Park and then has a healthy breakfast. He is in great shape and has no pain. He knows he's a lucky guy. "I thank God every morning that I am still here and feeling great," he says with glee. "So many of my friends are gone and I'm still here." He spends his days talking to his sons and grandkids. Working toward his new goal, he enlisted the services of a speaker's bureau and hopes to give talks on his life to inspire others. He's become a YouTube celebrity from his recent talk to the US Navy. And he delivers not only a great story but does so with a sense of humor. When going through his list of military accomplishments, he says: "With all the braids on my dress uniform, I could get a job as a doorman."

Among all his life accomplishments, he is most proud of living a good life. "I'm very proud that I've maintained my moral compass through life. I never compromised on what was important to me and my family and never deviated from my goals." If Mendes can still set goals at ninety-seven, so should everyone. Still a Marine through and through, he ends our conversation with "Semper fi." Do or die.

James Austin

DOB: August 31, 1942

Residences: Oaxaca, Mexico; Boston, Massachusetts; and Martha's
Vineyard, Massachusetts

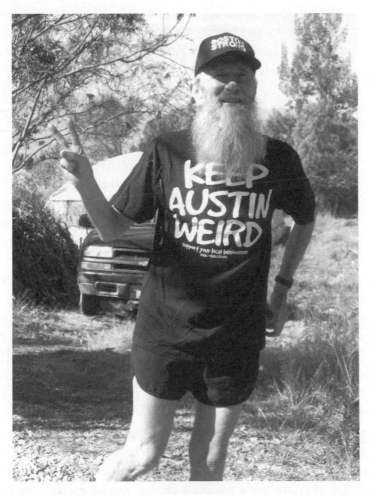

Jim Austin

"Travel the world and encounter animals large and small."
Most runners know that the best way to get around a new destination
is to run it. From early morning runs to spot the best breakfast venue or
exploring a new city, its parks and interesting sights, running is the way
to go. Jim Austin knows about these spots and more. In his book, *Gone
Running*, Austin says: "Discovery is the gift of exploring, and running
often leads you to explore nooks and crannies that otherwise would go
unseen, particularly when you find yourself in a new place. Trotting along
and taking whatever turn occurs to you can pull back the curtain and let
you see things that never would have been noticed zipping along in a
car." A runner for more than fifty years, Austin got his start in running
to escape schoolyard bullies in sixth grade. In his ever-present, humorous
style, he explains that he was too small and scrawny for football and ended
up breaking his arm. He tried basketball but was again too scrawny and
ended up breaking his arm. He tried weight lifting but in a gym session
lifting weights to build his scrawny body, he broke his arm. He swam on
his high school and college swim teams but wasn't very powerful in the
pool. But it turned out that scrawny body was just right for running.

While doing graduate work at Harvard in 1968 he ran his first
marathon, Boston. There were no qualifying times then and a record
high of 1,014 runners started out at Hopkinton. With little training
and no plan, he finished in three hours and seven minutes. It took him
twenty years to run his second marathon, the 1988 New York City Marathon, finishing in two hours and fifty-seven minutes. With a coveted
sub-three-hour marathon under his belt he thought he was done with
marathons but then the one-hundredth Boston loomed in 1996 so he
laced up his marathon shoes once more and finished in three hours and
twenty minutes. While Jim had completed his marathon trilogy, his son-
in-law Jose followed in his footsteps. This included running the Boston
Marathon to raise money for the Martin Richards Foundation and to
honor Martin, the youngest victim of the Boston Marathon bombing
and a playmate of Jose and, Jim's daughter, Amy's children.

On a trip to the Galapagos with his grandchildren, he ran and
swerved through hundreds of sunbathing sea lions. On a trip to Botswana,
where his wife Cathy was collaborating with a women's micro-finance
organization, they went on a safari. Warned not to go running outside
of the camp unless he could run faster than a lion, he promised to stay
close to the perimeter of the camp. His run was going well until he

ran full tilt into a herd of charging elephants. "As I am coming back to camp, I suddenly feel the ground trembling. *An earthquake?* I thought. I look around to see a herd of elephants running full tilt in my direction," he recalls. "I had visions of a squashed Austin flashing in my head." The elephants were headed for a watering hole and luckily for Austin had no interest in him.

On a fishing trip to Alaska with his brother and two sons, he had a close encounter with a grizzly bear. They booked a lodge on the Cooper River, famous for its salmon fishing and hungry grizzly bears. Having grown up in Michigan, family fishing vacations to nearby Canada were a tradition. They flew in on a float plane and then took jet boats to the lodge. The guide gave them explicit instructions to stay away from the bears and never, ever, come between a mother bear and her cub. Austin was barred from running the trails around the lodge and was relegated to using an elliptical machine. One morning, already bored with the elliptical, he popped his head outside thinking, *maybe I can outrun a bear*. Then he heard a startling sound and on the banks of the river stood a male grizzly at full height roaring and waving its arms as if to attack. After that the elliptical seemed like a good idea.

Then there were the bats in Lahore, Pakistan. While advising a new university on its management school program, Austin heard about a 140-acre park. Leaving at dawn, he ran to the main gates of the park and suddenly heard a whooshing sound. Looking up, he saw hundreds of enormous bats with five-foot wing spans swooping down on him. As visions of vampire bats danced in his head, Austin ducked and then realized they are landing in the trees, not his head. Turns out they were giant fruit bats, not blood-sucking vampire ones. But just in case, he bolted back to the hotel.

While going to a conference in Barcelona, Jim was invited by Cathy to take the week beforehand and walk a portion of the famed Camino de Santiago, a ritualistic pilgrimage in northwestern Spain, a five-hundred-mile journey Cathy had completed before. This piece of the Camino was from Burgos to Astorga, 160 miles; roughly a fifteen-mile-a-day hike, Austin ended each day with a run through the local villages where they were greeted with "*Buen Camino, peregrino*" (travel well, pilgrim). Walking the Camino was a spiritual experience for Austin.

On the last day of the journey, Cathy realized she had lost her sunglasses. Austin absurdly said that he will run back to search for them somewhere along their route. He headed out and tried to retrace his steps, only to get lost as he ran in the opposite direction and so missed the trail signs. To make matters worse, it started to rain. But then he sees a hawk circling overhead and knows everything will turn out. "The sight of the hawk sharpened my concentration. I know it was a sign sent from St. James," he declared. "I started searching under bushes, a planting of small fir trees that Cathy had stopped to admire but nada, no glasses. I asked a passing young couple if they saw glasses and they just stared at this bearded loco in running shorts and a singlet in the rain and quickly moved on. An inner force urged me on, but I decided to turn around before it got dark. The hawk returned, and as I swung my head to see him, I caught a glimpse of an eyeglass cleaning cloth and there were the glasses." As he likes to say, "A pilgrim can leave the Camino, but the Camino never leaves the Pilgrim."

Having visited Machu Picchu, the Lost City of the Incas in the Peruvian Andres, in 1966, Austin always wanted to return. In November of 2010 his wish was granted when he received an invitation to Peru from the Universidad del Pacífico to receive an honorary professorship in management. This time, he was gung-ho on hiking the original Inca trails to the ancient city rather than take the train. He was uncertain how his sixty-seven-year-old body would react to the higher altitude on the four-day trail journey that starts at 9,000 feet, climbs to 13,700 feet, and then descends and rises again before descending down to Machu Picchu. The total distance is about the same as a marathon, but the terrain is treacherous.

He flew into Cusco to start the four-day hike and immediately got hit with an altitude headache. He sipped mate de coco, the local tea, took a Dioxin pill, and tried to sleep. Early the next morning, before starting the hike, he bought a collapsible walking stick that he declared the best $12 investment he ever made. His guide, Leo, was a runner. The first day's hike was rocky and hard to trot in some areas, but Austin kept chugging away. He started to pass other porters and trekkers and was feeling good, especially when a porter he passes yelled out, *Fuerte, Fuerte*! (Strong, strong!). Around the campgrounds that night, the other guides asked Leo if he is guiding Forrest Gump.

The second day was perilous, ascending to 13,776 feet, higher than he has ever been before. The trail was not only steep but rocky and tough on his already fragile ankle. He wrote: "Climbing up has been demanding in terms of exertion, but it is much more perilous descending on the slippery rock steps." The trail was the original one used from the sixth century. They cut the day short due to the slippery rocks and the cold. "I bundled up in thermal underwear and socks and remain toasty warm," he recalls.

Day three was the longest trek and started with a steep one-mile ascent at 12,400 feet. The views were exhilarating and the climb invigorating. At the end of the day, Austin's trotting strong, which surprised his porter, Manuel. He asked if Austin races and he replied in the affirmative. Manuel raced as well, and his younger brother, also a runner, won the Inca Trail Marathon in the 1990s. Austin was impressed with the running lineage. That night, their last before entering the ancient city, Austin prepared himself for the final step of the journey.

Day four, the final day before entering the city, Austin was particularly stoked. His goal was to be the first visitor to enter the control station when it opens at 5:30 a.m. They rose at 2:45 and arrived at Machu Picchu with the sun just coming over the mountain tops, its rays spotlighting Machu Picchu in gold, framed by the mountain shadows.

Despite his world travels, Austin's favorite race is in his backyard, the Martha's Vineyard Chilmark Road Race 5K. What started as a local fundraiser in 1978 with 180 entrants has grown into a sold-out race with 1,600 runners. He has run it with his spouse, sons, daughter, son-in-law, and grandchildren.

Now seventy-five, Austin knows his fast running days are in the past. "My conversations with fellow runners my age center on our injuries," he laughs. He underwent ankle surgery at sixty-nine to remove a spur and perform microfracture chondroplasty. His surgeon said to him, "Most people in this situation would find another activity but I understand you are a committed runner." Austin likes to add that what the doctor implied is that committed runners were not normal. Seven months after the surgery he ran a five-miler, his slowest race ever, but he edges out another geezer at the finish to take third in his age group. As he wisely states, "Speediness is in the eyes of the beholder."

"I don't start in the front anymore now that I am a mid-pack runner," he says. "Accepting the fact that your machine just isn't the same anymore is psychologically wrenching. But it is what it is and at least I am still running. You just have to reconcile yourself to getting slower, which is hard to take for some runners who can't stop looking in the rearview mirror at previous years' times."

Austin doesn't have time to look in his rearview mirror. He's too busy traveling the world and running in exotic places, happy to share the experience with anyone who comes along.

Jamie and Lynn Parks

DOB: Jamie, December 12, 1961; Lynn, September 29, 1962

Residence: Tinley Park, Illinois

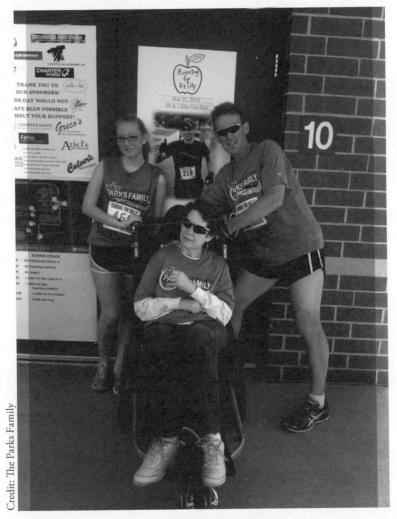

Annalyn, Lynn, and Jamie Parks

For Love.

In 2007, while writing for *Runner's World*, I had the pleasure of meeting Jamie and Lynn Parks and their daughter Annalyn. Their story was selected for the "Heroes" coverage in the December issue. It's a story of devoted love with running at its core.

Jamie and Lynn met at a party that neither of them had planned to attend. Jamie was a mail carrier, and Lynn was going to college. After just two months of dating, they were engaged. Then, five months before their wedding date, Lynn was involved in a car crash and suffered a brainstem injury that left her cognitively impaired, unable to walk, and not expected to live. She was in a coma for seventeen days. Jamie was told to prepare for the worst, but Lynn pushed through. When she was able to speak, she told Jamie she would marry him when she could walk down the aisle.

Jamie waited for the woman he loved for seven years, and in 1994, Lynn walked that short distance down the aisle to exchange their wedding vows. An avid runner, Jamie took Lynn to his races, leaving her at the start so she could see him but he always felt badly that he left her there. Inspired by Dick and Richard Holt, a father-and-son team that run the Boston Marathon with Dick pushing his son, who has cerebral palsy, in a wheelchair, Jamie started pushing her in races in 1991.

"I am so lucky Jamie has given me this gift," Lynn says. The fifty-six-year-olds have covered more than 27,500 miles together. Their personal bests include a 17:35 5K and a 2:57 at the 1996 Chicago Marathon. Pretty amazing times considering the weight Jamie pushes. (Lynn and the chair combined weigh 170 pounds.)

"She faces so many challenges but never complains," says Jamie. "It makes it hard for me to complain about anything." At a half marathon in August of 2003, one of the chair's wheels fell off at mile 12. Jamie pushed Lynn on a single wheel for the final mile, finishing in 1:32:11. "We were mad, but then you have to move on," Jamie says. "We don't take things as seriously as other folks might. Our big picture is much bigger."

In 1999, Lynn defied all odds again and had a baby girl, Annalyn. After her accident, her doctors advised her not to get pregnant, as she most likely would not be able to carry the baby to full term. Chalk up another miracle for the Parks family. Annalyn joined her parents at the races sitting in Lynn's lap. "We did run fifty-three races and a total of 4,051.1 miles with her," says a proud Jamie. "By age four she was on her own, old enough to do races herself."

After their recognition in 2007 as *Runner's World* "Heroes," their story caught the attention of A Step Ahead Prosthetics and Orthotics, who offered to design and create a racing chair for Lynn. Aided by the upgraded wheels and customized chair, the pair competed in the 2008 Boston Marathon, finishing in 3:25. Their story and training for Boston were filmed for a documentary featuring Lynn and Jamie called *Marathon Love*, which has won several film-festival awards. The pair has spoken at race expos in the United States.

They compete in Jamie's age category, never in a wheelchair division, and have won several races outright. In 2002, they carried the Olympic torch through Chicago on its way to the Winter Olympics in Salt Lake City, Utah.

For Jamie, it isn't enough to push his wife in races. He started a running streak in January of 1992, running a mile a day and has upheld that streak for twenty-six years and counting. He had a medical emergency last year that almost derailed his streak. He was on a training run pushing Lynn in the wheelchair. He was short of breath and found he had to slow down going up a slight incline and "felt like I was climbing a mountain," he recalls. As he started back home, fatigued, he had trouble breathing. The rest of the day he felt a fluttering in his heart, which continued into to the next day. He went to the emergency room, where an EKG was taken. Seeing the results, the doctor sent him immediately to the hospital realizing he was suffering from atrial fibrillation. He was kept in the hospital overnight for observation and he wondered how he was going to get his streak in unnoticed by the nurses and doctors who had ordered rest. He measured the circumference of his hospital room and at night when no one was looking, ran a mile in his room back and forth to the bathroom. The streak was safe.

A chip off the old block, Annalyn started her own running streak at age nine and ended it at seventeen when she needed to dedicate more time to college preparatory courses. Now a freshman in college, she is training to be a pastry chef. She's quite an accomplished runner in her own right running her first half marathon at age thirteen in 2:11:58.

The Parks recently completed their sixth marathon together at the 2018 Boston Marathon in what has been hailed as the worst weather ever. They drove to Boston in their new thirty-two-foot RV and parked in a town close to Hopkinton. "It was miserable," laments Jamie. "After the first three miles I told Lynn we were not going to race but hunker down to just finish the darn thing." Lynn was dressed in five layers but remained cold throughout due to the driving winds and rain. Jamie wore rain gear but his shoes and socks were soaked and his two layers of gloves didn't keep his hands warm as he pushed the wheelchair, which accumulated added weight due to the rain and extra clothing. The initial plan was to enjoy the race and high-five friends along the course, but that plan deteriorated along with the weather. "I'm very competitive and this was our slowest race time ever," states Jamie with disappointment tinged in his voice. At the finish, Lynn's first words were, "no more marathons!" Three months later, keeping his word, Jamie and Lynn competed in a July Fourth 5K close to home.

Now retired from the postal service after thirty-seven years, Jamie will have more time to dedicate to Lynn and their common love of running together. But not one to sit around, Jamie became an Uber driver in September of 2017 in anticipation of using it as a supplemental income after retirement. Lynn sometimes accompanies him on his rides. "We both love to meet people and talk, so this is a fun job that works out for both of us," says Jamie. The customers seem to agree as they become enthralled by their story and don't want to get out of the car.

This is a love story with running at its core. An accomplished runner, Jamie could run faster on his own, as some have told him. That's not his goal. He lives to run and to run with Lynn. "Our love has been set in stone since the day we met," says Jamie. "After thirty-three years of marriage, I find I want to spend even more time with Lynn, not less." Jamie gets reflective of their years together looking forward: "Part of the reason I retired at age fifty-six is to spend more time with Lynn. I have friends who waited 'til retirement to spend more time with their spouses and then something tragic happens and those golden-year plans are never shared. I want to grow old with Lynn."

Jamie and Lynn have a strong sense of faith that has helped pull them through their difficult times. When they give their talk at race expos, some people question how they could still have faith with everything that happened to Lynn. Jamie responds: "I could curse God for that car crash and letting her suffer, but I can also thank God for letting her live and being my wife and partner all these wonderful years." Their strong faith and a twisted sense of humor keep the Parks rolling through life and marathons.

Lessons Learned

Nurture the Gift

There are so many takeaways from the runners interviewed for this book that it's difficult to find a starting point for all the lessons learned. What comes across loud and clear from every runner, regardless of age or level of running, is that running is a gift to be nurtured and treasured. Everyone wants to run forever, to pursue endless miles until they can't. The wonderful and inspiring Toshiko d'Elia, who is one of my role models, used to tell me to take care of my running like a close friend. "Never disrespect your running or take it for granted," she advised.

She was very wise. After a race the first thing she did, after she had a cold beer, was to thank her feet. The first time she did this I was a bit amazed. She sat on the floor in our hotel room and massaged her feet, thanking them for carrying her through the race. She soothed every toe and massaged her soles. It was a very Zen-like act but one I adopted as a way of taking care of my feet, a way of nurturing the gift.

Gordon Bakoulis said: "I get as much as I give from the sport that I love so much. I plan to preserve this gift for as long as I can." That's probably the most important lesson for every runner but especially for those of us who are at an age where we can see the final finish line. Cherish the time you have with your running. Japanese writer and runner Haruki Murakami's 2007 memoir, *What I Talk About When I Talk About Running*, is a bit of a cult book that should be a must-read for all runners. He has a view of running that is inseparable from his life: "First there came the action of running, and accompanying it there was this entity known as me. I run; therefore I am." Nurture your running and in return it will take care of you.

Don't Forget Where You Came from

Many of the people I interviewed are part of the Greatest Generation, a term popularized by Tom Brokaw's 1998 book of the same name. It's defined as people who grew up during the Depression and went on to fight in World War II. Brokaw aptly describes that: "These men and women developed values of personal responsibility, duty, honor, and faith in a humble manner." Many of the Greatest Generation runners I interviewed grew up poor, on a farm, working hard from the age of four. Charles Milliman grew up during the Depression and his family didn't know where the next meal would come from. To this day, he never throws anything out. He credits his work ethic at an early age with his ability to run eighty-five miles on his eighty-fifth birthday. Jonathan Mendes thinks nothing of run/walking a marathon at age ninety-six and celebrating with a glass of scotch. He flew fighter planes in the war. Running a marathon is just another challenge for him, and he is up for the task.

If you are younger than that generation, you're a baby boomer, starting with a birth date of 1946. Baby boomers are also pretty resilient. Growing up in the late forties and fifties left a mark of defiance on many. Whether protesting wars or fighting for women's rights, baby boomers are not silent. They are not afraid to question the establishment and are goal-oriented and resourceful. They are change-makers who went into the Peace Corps after college, like James Austin or Julia Chase who helped change the rules governing the distance women were allowed to compete in by breaking the rules. Running is an activity that appeals to their sense of social community and grassroots organizations. Runners like Drew Swiss, who runs to raise money for under-privileged kids, never forgets where he came from and the struggles of growing up with bad eating habits that caused him to be overweight and bullied as a kid. Alisa Harvey is thankful for everything her parents did for her growing up with financial struggles and did her best in her track career to make them proud of her. "I wanted to do well for me and my family. My parents didn't get to go to college and gave me the emotional support to train hard to get here, and I wanted them to be proud," she says.

Many of the octogenarians and beyond that I spoke with tell me what they have witnessed in their lifetime. Julia Hawkins has seen the invention of airplanes, televisions, cell phones, men landing on the moon, and more during her lifetime. If you ask her if any of these inventions have changed her life, she'll tell you the biggest impact on her life is her family and feeling needed and loved. "At 102, my hands don't always do what I tell them to do and my mind doesn't click along like it used to," she states. "But I have my four wonderful children, grandchildren, and now a great-child, and that is all the purpose in the world I need." Hawkins has never forgotten where she came from or that every day of her life shaped her into becoming a world-record holder.

Whatever your background, use it and turn to it for inspiration. It's a part of your DNA. Many non-runners like to ask, "What are you running from?" Most of us are not running away from something but running to something. We are running to a better lifestyle, new experiences, and endless possibilities. The road beckons us.

Fight the Stereotype of Old Age

Masters runners are changing the way society views old age and its negative pervasive stereotypes. At eighty, Gerry Miller is as young at heart as anyone half his age. His advice: "Stay positive, enjoy life, have the odd beer. As we get older, we don't have to run but we have to keep moving because physically moving kind of helps one to stay active mentally and intellectually as well. All variables come together—if we eat well, we move, we stay positive, we keep our life's vibrations as high as possible." Or as Ken Stone says, "We have earned the right to do whatever we want."

Sportswriter and coach Marc Bloom has been running since he was in high school in Sheepshead Bay, Brooklyn, and has been covering track and field since about the same time. "I've been around a long time," says Bloom. Now seventy, he knows his PRs are behind him but that doesn't stop him from competing and being the best he can be. Which is still pretty fast. In 2017, at age seventy, he clocked 6:16 at the Fifth Avenue Mile.

Bloom has been coaching girls and boys track and cross country at Hillsborough High School in New Jersey for five years. He feels he has learned a lot from running with high school kids and it has given him a new appreciation for running. "They are who I want to be now, at seventy!" he states. "I want the mind and outlook of a teenager. There's no feeling like running with a bunch of teenagers who are striving towards a level of excellence." Bloom feels that we can all learn from their spirit and youth and exuberance. "Their attitude is what helps to make me a better runner as I age." Bloom advises to never give a thought to your age or how you should behave.

Betty Lindberg was a self-described couch potato until sixty-three. Now ninety-three, she feels like a kid and does whatever she wants. She knows how to navigate her cell phone like a teenager and drives herself around Atlanta to get to the Apple store or her workouts with the Atlanta Track Club. At seventy-eight, Kathy Bergen loves to sit around the track with her girlfriends and talk about meets, records, and who is entering a new age group. Discovering masters track at age fifty-four changed her life and allowed her to be the athlete she always wanted to be but the pre-Title IX era barred her from many high school sports. Her grandchildren think she is a hoot and love that fact that she is so active and younger in mind and body than most grandmas.

Anti-aging? I used to embrace that term and was a sucker for all the anti-aging products that flooded the market. A cream that will erase wrinkles? I bought lots of them. But the only thing that disappeared was the cash in my wallet. I bought life extension vitamins to rejuvenate my cells but I don't think my cells got any younger. According to an article in *Time* magazine, anti-aging products from skin creams to chemical peels are part of a $250 billion worldwide industry, but scientists have yet to discover a longevity elixir that stands up to medical scrutiny. Physicist Julian Gordon said it succinctly: "Anyone can define a term and use it for whatever rubbish they might think fit. But anti-aging that promises to reverse aging is at the best puffery, at the worst fraud. I don't think aging can be reversed. The best thing to do is to maintain vigorous physical and mental health to minimize the effects of aging." As runners, we know what that elixir is. It's running. Instead of the term anti-aging, embrace the term positive-aging.

The cliché that age is just a number might be beaten to death but it is so true. According to a study of aging from the University of Michigan and the Max Planck Institute for Human Development in Berlin, older people feel, on average, about thirteen years younger than they really are. So seventy is the new fifty-seven. Among study participants who were particularly healthy and active, the gap between subjective age and actual age was even wider. The data are important because cultural expectations of people during their older years often are at odds with how seniors perceive themselves. Think of the birthday cards of screeching old women or men in rocking chairs. That is not us. Dr. Jacqui Smith, a psychologist at the University of Michigan Institute for Social Research said, "If you self-define yourself as someone who is old, then you probably act that way." So better to act like Betty Lindberg, Kathy Bergen, or Gerry Miller. Next time it rains, go for a run and splash in the puddles like you are a kid again. Or hop on a bike like 102-year-old Julia Hawkins and take a spin around the neighborhood. Or think like Harold Green who wakes up every morning with this thought: "Life is a precious commodity. All we have is time and our health. Savor it."

Embrace the Running Community

Throughout my interviews, every runner I spoke with talked about the importance of being part of the fabric of a supportive community. George Hirsch looks forward to seeing friends once a year at running events and catching up with their lives. Tom Perri meets up with runners he has paced at marathons and they sign up to be paced with him again because they love his spirit, his positive energy, and he gets them to their target time. Attending races, which he does almost every weekend, is his way of staying socially connected. Runners also pointed out the unconditional support and loyalty of the running community. We cheer as loudly for the first-place finisher as we do the last-place finisher. At the New York Road Runner's Mini 10K, the world's original women-only road race, the course is lined with fathers, husbands, sons, and male club members cheering for the female runners, their mothers, wives, girlfriends, and grandmothers. Peter Ciaccia, race director of the New York City Marathon, waits until the last runner crosses the finish line and gives them the same greeting as the elites who finished upwards of eleven hours earlier. He says it's his favorite part of the race. Bill Rodgers loves the way running has evolved into an Everyman's sport, so different from when he was running competitively. "It's no longer just the fast and fittest who attend races," he states. "It's families, it's girlfriends and boyfriends, first-timers and old timers. That's the beauty of our sport, that everyone feels welcome."

On most weekends I can drive into New York City and line up for an NYRR race that on average has more than 2,000 runners. I am always astounded that on Saturday morning that many people are ready to run. It's like a party. I always find someone I know and spend time catching up, warming up, or talking in the port-a-potty line. It's a feel-good way to start the day. And afterward there are invites to brunch and discussions of the next race to come. It's a special community that embraces all comers.

Marc Bloom states about running: "I strongly endorse the value of a support system that includes fellow runners of any age who provide a communal spirit, motivation, and comradeship." Bill Gross called me back after our interview to ask if he could add something about the importance of the running community. He told me: "Being a runner is like being a member of a tribe. We are a bunch of like-minded individuals drawn together by a shared passion. We travel from town to town to participate in a precisely measured event. It is the passion that draws us together regardless of age."

Gross raises the importance of the age difference for a reason. "Our age differences enhance the tribe. I watch older runners finding ways to calm down the younger, jittery, first-timers. We older runners are motivated by the fresh enthusiasm and contagious energy of younger runners," he adds. I have fond memories of traveling to races with my female race buddies, including Toshi. As the youngest member of the tribe of traveling runners, I was the designated driver. In long car rides I would listen to their stories of running the Boston or New York City Marathons back in the day. We shared rooms together and again being the youngest, I slept on the floor. We learned each other's race habits and rituals and were sworn to secrecy about who needed an enema before a race. We were a community of runners and friends, and we showed the utmost respect for each other, supported each other and cheered for each other. Sometimes you don't get that from immediate family members but you can always count on your running buddies.

Linda Cohn is that late-blooming athlete who found a new life when she turned fifty and started attending the Huntsman Senior Games in Utah, describing it as "a fulfillment of my dreams since I was a kid." Her first experience at the Games altered her life's path forever. "The Games sparked a desire to see where track and field could take me, and has allowed me to travel the world to compete and become a world champion," states Cohn. "Track and field is a pretty individual sport. We each have our own events and personal goals. However one thing has become very clear to me especially when I've had the opportunity to run relays. Track is so much more fun when you are a member of a team."

Running can be a solo pursuit and many of us cherish our time alone on the road or path. But don't miss out on the opportunity to be a part of this magical community that understands us. Who else wants to hear our running and racing stories for the umpteenth time? Runners do.

Be Fearless

I have to thank Kathrine Switzer for first using the word fearless to describe how running makes us feel. Switzer used it to describe how running makes women feel, but I heard it in the voices of the men I interviewed as well. Fearless can mean many things but it can also mean not caring about what others think. Getting past fifty is so freeing in many ways. Who cares what people say or how we look or how we act. So over that. Run when many non-running folks think we are too old to put on running shorts and a singlet and sweat? You bet!

As runners over fifty we are also changing the face of aging in our society. As Bob Lida stated so well, "It's easy to give in to feeling old and acting old because that's how our society sees us." We need to change that. Walk up the stairs instead of taking the escalator. Practice balance exercises every day so we don't have to rely on a cane or walk stooped. Act how you feel, not your age.

Be Inspired

One of the things that I loved about writing this book is the inspiration I felt after completing each interview. I felt renewed, young, and ready to go for a run. How could I not want to go for a run after talking with Kathy Martin? I'll never be as fast as her but she inspires me to do my best. I see her at the races (always from the rear) and I know how hard she trains. Although that's not my goal, it's a reminder to never give up. Ed Rousseau's straight talk about his alcoholism was also inspiring. He acknowledges his addiction and wants to help others. He uses running as a way to stay sober. As he states, "I substituted another mile for another drink." His dedication to staying sober and healthy for over thirty years is more than impressive.

On days that I might have been feeling a bit lazy to get out the door on a run, I would review my stories and focus on Mike Brooks who runs through snow, ice, back issues, and sore knees. I don't advocate everything Brooks does, but he is inspiring. I also got a laugh from streaker Brian Salzberg who completed the Falmouth Road Race on crutches one year to keep the streak alive. One runner I didn't cover in this book but have known for years is Irapaul Turner. I met Irapaul on his first day of training for the New York City Marathon back in 2012. He had joined Team for Kids (TFK) when I was coaching. We all remember Irapaul, a gentle giant of a man who approached us with trepidation about learning to run. At over six feet and weighing 340 pounds, he thought we would tell him to go home, that he could never run a marathon. In that instant, he won our hearts with his determination and drive to succeed. His first marathon was not a success story. He fell coming down the ramp of the Queensborough Bridge at mile 16 and had to be taken to the hospital. As he puts it: "I was a big black ball tumbling down to agony and the end of my marathon dream." But he came back the next year and the next and has now run twelve marathons in four years. He's lost 125 pounds and in April of 2018, at age fifty, ran the Boston Marathon as a fundraiser for TFK. Not only did he run the most iconic marathon in the world, when he finished, he collected the Abbot World Majors Medal. Boston was the keystone of his four-year journey to collect the medal. To this day, when any of the TFK coaches see him, he thanks us for allowing him to run with us. But Irapaul has it all wrong. His humbleness and determination and staunch belief that he will run a marathon is what makes him a runner, not our coaching. "Running changed my life and gave me lifelong friends," says a grateful Turner.

Pay It Forward

As a community, runners support one another through thick and thin. When a runner is kind and supportive to you, pass it on to the next runner. The best example of this I can recall is the time I raced the 2004 Cherry Blossom 10 Miler in DC. I had a goal in mind and within the first mile tucked in behind a man who was running just slightly faster than my goal pace. I stayed right behind his left shoulder for nine and a half miles. With half a mile to go he picked up the pace and started sprinting to the finish. I was pretty much shot at that point and couldn't keep up. I started to drift back when suddenly his left hand shot out and grabbed me. He pulled me next to him saying, "We've been together for nine miles darlin' and I'm not letting you go now." How did he know I was there? I never bumped him or spoke to him. He held my hand till just before we crossed the finish line and my PR, and then he dropped it, fading into the crowd as he finished. After I caught my breath I searched for him but never saw him again. I call him my Running Angel.

I've also played a Running Angel. At a race in Central Park I was shooting for a specific time. I ran my butt off, but when I finished, I missed my target time. Like an obsessed runner, I started kicking myself and rehashing the race. "Should have picked it up at mile 3. Shouldn't have taken water at mile 5," and so on. In the middle of my silent tirade I felt a tap on my shoulder and turned to see another runner. "I just want to thank you for pacing me to a PR today. I ran behind you the entire race and you kept the pace I needed." With that I got a sweaty hug and the dude moved on. You never know whom you are pulling along or who is pushing you to succeed. Just be thankful and keep on pushing and pulling.

Another lesson I learned is to always thank the volunteers on the course. They've been there since the crack of dawn or earlier in all kinds of weather. Every time I pass a volunteer, I thank them. Just a quick "thanks for being here." It only takes a second. It makes me feel good to thank the people who put on the race because without them we wouldn't have a race.

Carpe Diem

There are many more lessons learned gleaned from these pages and through the voices and thoughts of the runners. Like Karen Bowler's belief to smile every day. "It's important to smile as it relaxes the face and makes everyone feel good. I spend a lot of time smiling. My life has been a wonderful journey and the best part is that it isn't over yet," says Bowler. Find one that resonates with you. And finally, the last word from Sid Howard on lessons learned: "Just be the best you can be at any age."

Advice from the Experts

Michael Conlon: Physical Therapist, Marathon Coach

Michael Conlon founded Finish Line Physical Therapy in 2006 to provide service and personal attention to clients who range from runners of all ages and abilities to anyone needing physical therapy. He received his bachelors of science in physical therapy from the Hogeschool Enschede in the Netherlands and has been a New York State licensed physical therapist since 1997. Conlon is recognized as a Fellow of Applied Functional Science (FAFS) through the Gray Institute. He has run twenty-five marathons and has completed the Lake Placid Ironman three times.

As the former coach for the New York City chapter of the Leukemia and Lymphoma's Team in Training program from 2002 to 2016, Conlon trained hundreds of runners, from beginners to advanced marathoners. In 2016, he was named the head coach of Team for Kids, a group of adult runners who raise funds to run the New York City Marathon and other major marathons and half-marathon races to support youth running and fitness programs for New York Road Runners.

I met Conlon when I was coaching Team for Kids. His engaging warmth, knowledge, and "can-do" attitude makes him a favorite with the team members.

Q: Do you treat older runners differently than younger runners who are training for a marathon?
A: We don't treat them any differently. A marathon is a marathon and everyone from twenty-five to eighty-five has to put in the miles. Having said that, I find that older runners are more compliant with the details of the training and more focused on doing things correctly. They are more

likely to do self-myofascial therapy (a.k.a. foam roll), stretch, and warm up before a run. They focus on the quality of their training and are very mindful of the things they can't do.

Q: What are some of the differences you see in training the younger runners versus the older ones?

A: The older runners know they aren't immortal. An injury could mean the end of their running and they don't ever want that to happen. They have a passion and respect for running that comes with maturity and more miles underneath their shoes. The younger runners tend to be like young bucks, thinking they are immortal and nothing will sideline them. They will run through an injury, which could make it worse, whereas the older ones will come in and get the injury treated right away.

Q: How do you feel about high-intensity training for older runners? Some coaches are advocating this training technique for the aging runner as opposed to the traditional LSD (long slow distance runs).

A: I don't necessarily advocate for high-intensity training for older athletes but instead prefer to have them focus on the quality of training versus the quantity of training. If a particular individual can handle more weekly "volume" in their schedule I would have them opt for non-impact cross-training (i.e. elliptical trainer) instead of adding more running volume to their training program.

Q: How are the muscles and fibers different in the older runners you treat and coach?

A: As we age, tissues become less elastic due to decreased collagen growth. The tissues also get dehydrated. Think of the difference between a grape and a raisin. Tissues ideally should be supple like a grape but as cellular development drops off during the aging process they become more like raisins, so the older runner has to hydrate more to get that suppleness. Soft tissue injuries will take longer to heal in aging runners as well, but the good news is that soft tissue injuries can heal.

Q: What do you recommend older runners do to avoid injuries and stay in good running shape?

A: I always educate my older clients on the importance of proper form and movement techniques. No matter how long they have been running, it's always good to get a gait analysis and have someone look at their form with fresh eyes. Then I concentrate on the following:

- Hip and glute strength: I have them do lunges and squats in all three planes of motion (just because you are older doesn't mean your biomechanics stop functioning in all three planes: sagittal, frontal, and transverse) but modified to their level and definitely using the right form and technique.
- Weight strengthening: I have them use lighter weights and more repetitions than I would with a younger runner.
- Flexibility (Mobility): Stretching/mobility becomes more important in older runners as tissues and muscles become tight. If the body stays flexible/mobile/stable (strength), anyone can do squats and lunges. I have a seventy-two-year-old client who can do pull-ups and modified burpees. It makes her feel young and as long as she does them correctly, then good for her. Exercise has no age limit if done properly.
- Preparation: I'm a big fan of warm-ups and cooldowns. A twenty-year-old may be able to go all out at the start of a run but the fifty-year-old should take a few warm-up laps or risk injury such as pulling a muscle. Muscle strength, the ability to generate force, declines dramatically in our late thirties and early forties, so we really have to warm up the muscles.
- Recovery: This is key for all runners but especially for aging athletes. Our bodies take longer to recover after a run or workout than when we were young. The most important part of any runners' training is recovery. And it becomes more important as we age.

Conlon adds his own perspective on aging: "At forty-five, I'm close to being in this book, not as a reference but as a statistic. My PRs are behind me and I am getting slower. But I get invigorated every day through my clients and the people I coach. They are a daily reminder that if we take care of our bodies and listen to what they are saying (or screaming) at us, we can all achieve endless miles.

"My goal as a physical therapist and a coach is to get my clients up and running. I try to get them to understand and own the fact that running is a high-impact and stressful sport, but if you treat it with respect, you can run for life. That means aging runners have to religiously warm up and cool down. I don't advise running seven days a week. My marathon training schedule for the teams I coach consists of five days of running, one day of cross-training, and one day of full rest. The ultimate goal is to keep moving."

Tony Ruiz: Coach, Central Park Track Club

Tony Ruiz has been head road coach of the Central Park Track Club (CPTC) in New York since 1987. He brings with him years of coaching experience since his first coaching job as a twenty-six-year-old for a girls' team in Brooklyn. He has trained masters-level runners, beginners, professionals, friends, and strangers.

Prior to his coaching position at CPTC, he was the assistant coach at Iona College in Manhattan where he received his BA. He also brings with him a stellar running career, starting at fourteen when he was a junior national champion in the 800. At nineteen, he was an alternate in the 800 and 1500 for the 1980 Olympics, which were boycotted by the United States. "I had an entire life of running at the highest level before I graduated from college," says Ruiz.

Ruiz brings a lot of passion to his coaching. Ruiz, fifty-seven, grew up in the projects of East New York in a tough neighborhood. If you weren't a member of a gang, you had no identity. For Ruiz, running was his outlet. "Running kept me out of trouble," he says. He knows firsthand the value and importance of running and loves passing that on to others.

His training techniques came from his mentors and reading every running book he could get his hands on. His overall approach is simple: 1) practice is key; 2) avoid overtraining; and 3) get your head in the game. CPTC has a lot of masters runners and Ruiz doesn't vary in his training for them but does do a few things differently for the sixty-plus age group, namely:

1. Less volume: If the overall workout includes a six-mile tempo run, I'll have the sixty-plus age group do four miles. If the overall workout includes twelve quarters, I'll tell them to run eight, and to do them slower.

2. Less intensity: If I give an overall workout of 8 x 200s, I'll tell the seniors to do 5 x 300 and run at speed but not a forceful speed that puts stress on the muscles.

3. Weekly workouts: I advise to do one hard workout and one speed workout a week.

4. Back off: If you feel you are pushing too hard, be smart and back off.

5. Warm-ups: Older runners need to loosen their muscles, which get tighter as they age, and get the proper warm-up in before a workout. I suggest a ten- to twelve-minute easy run at conversation pace, just enough to loosen the muscles and raise the heart rate.

6. Warm-up drills: All runners but especially the older ones need to do dynamic stretching to gives your muscles, bones, and joints a chance to loosen up. Gradually bring up your heart rate and get into the rhythm you want to sustain. Incorporate the following into your warm-up drills: high knees, butt kicks, strides, etc.

7. Conditioning: Exercising all muscle groups becomes more important as you age. The hips, lower back, and upper body need to be conditioned and toned.

8. Balance: The older we get the more that balance becomes important. I stress to my older runners that they do balance exercises like standing on one leg when they brush their teeth.

9. Run on a soft surface: When possible run on grass or a soft-packed trail or track. Stay off the roads to reduce the pounding.

It bothers him that some of masters runners who are competitive have a difficult time adjusting to losing their speed. He advises them to reset their goals and look forward to age-group placement or look at their age-graded percentile. "Every five years you get to be the baby in the group," he laughs. Ruiz enjoys working with masters. "I can see the passion in their eyes and they never give up," he says. "Runners form a brotherhood like I never experienced in any other sport. We're all different and run different paces but at the end of the day we care about each other and pull together for each other."

Dr. Andrew Rosen: Orthopaedic Surgeon, Upper East Orthopaedics, Manhattan, New York

Dr. Andrew Rosen trained in Orthopaedic Surgery at Mount Sinai Medical Center in New York followed by a fellowship in Sports Medicine and Knee Reconstruction at the Insall-Scott-Kelly Institute at Beth Israel Medical Center. He is the author of numerous scientific articles and book chapters on his specialty and is a sought-after speaker at medical educational conferences. With fifteen marathons under his belt and a PR of 2:58 at Berlin at age forty-three, Dr. Rosen has the knowledge and first-hand experience to work the medical tent of the New York City Marathon taking care of the elite athletes.

I have known Dr. Rosen for years through my work at New York Road Runners. He was my go-to speaker for our marathon runners, giving humorous lectures on injury prevention and what to do when one occurs. On a personal level, Dr. Rosen has talked me off the ledge regarding my own injuries. I call him frantic and bewildered and he calms me down and if needed, prescribes a non-invasive treatment that gets me back to running.

Here is the Q&A with Dr. Rosen on injury prevention.

Q: What are the most common injuries you see in runners over fifty? Are they different? More frequent than younger runners?
A: There are commonalities in all runners, but the younger runners have more malalignment (incorrect or imperfect alignment) issues such as IT band and runner's knee because they are younger and haven't adapted their bodies to the rigors of running like the more seasoned runners. I see arthritis in the older ones, especially in the knees (but not in all runners) and more muscle strains such as in the calf and hamstring. At fifty-two, the body can't absorb the stress of pounding like a twenty-two-year-old.

Q: What are the effects of aging on a runner?
A: In general older runners have less of an ability to maintain aggressive training without risking injury. At fifty-five, you shouldn't be putting in the high mileage that you could when you were younger. As we age the body loses the ability to heal fast, so you end up with an overuse injury if you don't pay attention and take off for a few days. If that happens, you're looking at eight to ten weeks of recovery time versus six to eight weeks. Increased mileage catches up at some point to an older runner.

Q: How do you know when muscle soreness is normal or something to be concerned about and stop running?
A: This is a difficult concept for runners, as we all perceive pain differently. If the pain is just an annoying muscle ache or a little soreness, that's normal and nothing bad. Also if the pain is symmetrical, say in both legs or

calves, then it's probably just muscle soreness. But if the pain is isolated in one area and gets worse instead of better, and gets more intense the more you run, than you need to take a few days off. Stop when something stays.

Q: Do you advise runners to cross-train?
A: Cross-training is key for injury prevention. I recommend that runners cross-train with biking, swimming, and I also would add one day of rest. Overuse in terms of training or weekly mileage can lead to injury so definitely add in a day of complete rest and a day of cross-training in the workout schedule.

Q: What other suggestions do you have to avoid injury?
A: I tell my patients to invest in a foam roller, and use it! I also suggest getting deep tissue massages from a recommended sports professional, and if a muscle ache isn't going away, see a physical therapist as the first line of defense. And learn to ice after a hard workout or a minor ache. It's the first line of defense.

Q: What's your best piece of advice to stay healthy?
A: Don't take your running for granted. Take care of it. As we age we need to accept that what we "want" to achieve and what we "can" achieve are two different things. Your experiences change but can still be rewarding.

At forty-eight, Dr. Rosen is already seeing his future as an aging runner and is taking care of himself in the same manner he prescribes to his older patients. He's accepting that his PRs are behind him but that doesn't stop him from wanting to challenge himself. "My running has fallen off due to aging so I have to reset the goals. When I turn fifty in two years I'll shoot for age-group wins or settle for beating a time from last year instead of twenty years ago."

Dr. Rosen has found the balance between being competitive and being smart and looks ahead to running forever. He sums up: "Don't look back, look ahead. That's the takeaway."

Dr. Robert Conenello: DMP, Orangetown Podiatry, Orangetown, New York

Dr. Rob is the only person I allow to touch my feet. A runner, he understands when I say something like, "It feels weird here, kind of tingly."

He got me to wear toe spreaders to help with my neuroma and administered acoustic shockwave therapy in my feet. Both techniques helped get me back to running without pain. He is also kind and compassionate and knows real suffering. He is a cancer survivor, having endured two years of treatment for Stage IV throat cancer. He ran the 2018 United NYRR Half Marathon in March, raising money for AKTIV, the cancer foundation started by Grete Waitz. Here is Dr. Rob's advice for taking care of our aging feet.

Q: How important is our feet to our overall well-being as runners?
A: Your feet absorb three times your body weight, more force during running than any other part of the body. They propel us, giving us the power to move. They can make our runs enjoyable and pain-free or miserable, with blister and cracks and damaged toenails.

Q: What happens to our feet as we age?
A: Feet become both longer and wider as we age because the tendons and ligaments lose elasticity. The skin under our feet, called the fat pads, also gets thinner as we age, which can lead to injuries if it isn't kept supple through self-massage.

Q: What are the most common foot injuries you see in the older population of runners?
A: I see a lot of overuse injuries in older runners. And because the skin is thinner as explained, I see more neuromas and metatarsal injuries.

Q: What do you recommend as good foot therapy for runners?
A: Consider self-massage either using your thumbs or a foot-roller (available at many running shops) to stimulate the foot muscles. Rolling two or three golf balls or even a rolling pin under your feet also works well. Also consider foot-strengthening exercises such as:

1. **Toe rises.** Standing with feet slightly apart, rise up on your toes twenty times. Rise up on the count of one, and lower on the count of two and three.
2. **Towel pulls.** Put a towel under your foot and pull at it with your toes for thirty seconds. This helps to strengthen the muscles in the toes.
3. **Toe grabs.** Grasp a pencil or marble with your toes.
4. **Toe yoga.** Yoga poses, such as child's pose, help to lengthen the shins and feet muscles. Tree or stork poses also help with overall balance.

Q: How important is replacing shoes and socks?
A: Very! The average life of most running shoes is 350 to 500 miles, but if you're a heavier or taller runner, or if your gait isn't smooth, you may need new shoes sooner. An ill-fitting shoe can lead to numerous injuries that run all the way up the leg and into the hips, areas that you may not even connect to the shoes. A wider toe box is helpful in older runners as our feet expand.

Replacing socks is something runners don't normally think about. We all know the rule to replace shoes (see above) but socks aren't usually tossed when they get holes. Socks that have no cushioning or have lost their fit and become loose and bagged out are one of the primary causes of blisters. Wet socks and cotton socks can also cause blistering. And socks that are labeled with an L and R for left or right foot have been sized to accommodate the big toe so follow the fit.

Q: What's the best way to deal with foot injuries and when should a runner take the step to see a podiatrist?
A: Rule number one: if you are limping, stop running and see a sports doctor. Rule number two: if an ache or pain doesn't go away in five days, see a doctor. Seek out a professional who knows and understands runners. Avoid going to a "doc in the box" or generalist. The best way to recover is through relative rest, which keeps you active but at the same time recovering. If you have to stop running, stay active through cross-training.

Closing Remarks

I'm so blessed to have running in my life. It's my best friend, my religion, my cure-all. Running pre-dates meeting my husband in high school, so it's been a part of my life longer than he has, which is now forty-four years of marriage. Running is my elixir for anything that goes wrong in my life, emotionally or physically. Having a bad day? Go for a run. Having a great day? Probably started out with a run. When I was diagnosed with cancer for the second time in 2001, I was lucky to catch it early. As I lay in my hospital room post-surgery, I was already plotting a marathon even as I heard the doctor tell me no running for six weeks. I snuck in a few runs around the block until a well-meaning neighbor snitched on me. But as a runner, I knew that running a marathon was the only way I would know I was cured. Four months after the surgery, I ran the East Lyme Marathon in Connecticut and felt like I had destroyed any lingering cancer cells that had dared stayed behind. Dr. Rob Conenello tells me a similar story about completing the 2018 United NYRR Half Marathon three years after recovering from Stage IV throat cancer. When he crossed the finish line he said, "Okay cancer, I'm saying goodbye to you. Your time is up."

Running has introduced me to some of my closest and dearest friends. For the first twenty years of my running life I was a solo runner. Maybe because I started running under the cover of darkness as a secret, but I never wanted to share my running with anyone. It was my private time to reflect. But the summer I decided to run my first marathon, I met Ellen Bellicchi. We were seawall neighbors in New London and our kids were close friends. I knew Ellen ran so I mentioned my marathon plans. She had just run her first and offered to train me. *Gulp*! I didn't know what to say or how to avoid running with her. What if we didn't mesh? What if she was faster, slower? What if it was awkward and affected our friendship? I finally agreed to an early morning run with trepidation.

Turns out that was one of the best decisions I made. From the first mile, we were in synch. Our foot strikes matched, the conversation flowed, and I wanted to run more miles with her. Over that summer we ran almost every day, forming a lifelong bond. We had our own secret running code. Instead of calling her on the phone to kvetch about life or the kids or husbands, I would say, "I need a ten-miler" and she would know what that meant. Or she would call me and say, "My mother-in-law is here. I need an eighteen-miler." We'd meet at the corner and run endless miles through the beach towns. On our way back we'd race the submarines coming up the Thames River from the Naval Submarine Base in Groton heading out of port before disappearing beyond Race Rock Lighthouse in Long Island Sound. Our cooldown ritual was swimming to a raft and lying there, exhausted but exhilarated. It would still be early morning and we often watched the sun's early rays beam off the water. Everything was still and peaceful until someone spotted us—usually her mother-in-law—calling us back to reality.

Running has also been my guide as I navigate through my senior years. Those of us fifty and beyond are among the first generation of runners and agers who want to stay active and healthy, run for life, and not hang out the "just retired" sign. I can't imagine my life without running. When I'm injured and have to take a recovery break, I get jealous when I see other runners on the road enjoying their run. Which is why I try not to get injured. I've slowed down a lot. At first that was difficult to accept, but with age comes a bit of wisdom and I know that to run for life I need to run smarter. So I've accepted the fact that I will run slower than anticipated and be happy that I am running in a race at all. Because for me it's like being at a rock concert. The excited runners, the pre-race jitters standing in the corral waiting for the start, the singing of the National Anthem, the bands along the course, then the sprint to the finish line and best of all is sharing the moment with other the runners, some of whom I know while some are strangers, but we all embrace at the finish. I've been to at least two races where the recording of the National Anthem broke down and without missing a beat, thousands of runners picked up the words and carried on with the song. It still gives me chills when I think of those moments.

And can we talk for just a minute about how beautiful our sport is? When I see a runner with a perfect form and kick, it's like poetry in motion, so fluid and powerful yet stealth-like at the same time. I actually watch the entire 26.2 miles of an Olympic marathon when it is televised. In 2004, when Deena Kastor took bronze in Athens, I ran (in place) with her in my living room for the entire course. My town of Ridgewood, New Jersey, has an excellent high school track and cross-country team and I love watching the kids run through town. The words from the coaches are always encouraging and positive, unlike other sports where you hear coaches screaming at kids. I watch them crest a particularly long hill and at the top the coach waits with cool watermelon slices. As the runners finish the hill, they clap for the next runner and so on until there is a supportive cluster of teammates cheering for the last runner. Watching this gives me hope that these kids will be good leaders someday.

My own family has given me a lot of running joy, watching nieces and nephews turn into runners. Many of them have run marathons. I've been able to share the road with them at races. We start together, then they take off, but at the end we have family post-race parties. When my niece Dana married Jamey Gifford, a Stanford University runner who was teammates with Ryan Hall, I organized a pre-wedding day 5K for the wedding party and guests. The customized race bibs had their wedding date and the T-shirts had their photos on them. We set up hydration tables with cups of champagne. The race ended on the beach and we held a finish line tape made of seaweed for the winner.

I have enjoyed writing this book and feel a bit sad that the process is over. I feel very connected to all the people I interviewed. They opened their lives to me and I learned so much from them. We spoke freely, openly, and honestly with each other. When you reach a certain age there's an earned privilege in speaking up about what's really on your mind. There are so many other inspiring runners over fifty that I could have profiled. I wish them all luck with their running and aging. Because they go hand in hand.

Senior Events

There are a variety of senior games to attend, both track and road, if you feel like a challenge or to just enjoy the camaraderie of like-minded runners. As sixty-seven-year-old Linda Cohn states: "Unlike a lot of runners who competed earlier in their lives, I started track and field at the age of fifty. I do not have memories of college 'glory days' that I can compare to my current performances. In my mind, my best throws, jumps, and running times are still ahead of me. With my focus on these goals I don't think of myself as getting older, I'm working towards getting better!"

For local races, look to your newspaper, running store, or various runner websites for a calendar of events.

USA Track and Field has a website with a roster of both state and national competitions.

World Masters Games (WMA), organized by the International Masters Games Association, offers competition and friendship regardless of age, gender, race, religion, or sport status around the globe.

The Huntsman World Senior Games, St. George, Utah
The Huntsman World Senior Games is the largest annual multi-sport event in the world for athletes aged fifty and older. The event takes place each October in St. George, Utah.

***

Amby Burfoot, http://www.100klifetimemiles.com. Tracking runners with 100,000 mile or more lifetime miles.

***

National Masters News & MastersRankings.com, a website dedicated to serving Masters Athletes and Masters Athletics.

***

Ken Stone's masterstrack.blog.

Bibliography/Further Reading

Amby Burfoot, *Run Forever* (Center Street, 2018)

Daniel Lieberman, *The Story of the Human Body: Evolution, Health, and Disease* (New York: Vintage, 2014)

Deena Kastor and Michelle Hamilton, *Let Your Mind Run* (New York: Crown Archetype, 2018)

George Banks, *History of the Marine Corps Marathon* (New York: Meyer and Meyer Sport, 2008)

James Austin, *Gone Running* (self-published, 2015)

Jeff Galloway, *Run Walk Run Method* (New York: Meyer and Meyer Sport, 2016)

Julia Hawkins, *It's Been Wondrous! A Centenarian's Memoir* (Baton Rouge: Model A Press, 2017)

Michael Brooks, *Badwater and Beyond: A Thousand Races, Places & Faces* (CreateSpace Independent Publishing Platform, 2018)

Haruki Murakami, *What I Talk About When I Talk About Running* (New York: Vintage International, 2009)

Acknowledgments

I should start by thanking everyone I have ever run with or talked to about running or who inspired me to be a better runner. Among the many are my brothers who inspired me to run around the block when girls were not allowed on a track or cross-country team and my first running partner, Ellen Bellicchi, who trained me for my first marathon. Toshiko d'Elia, who took me under her wing and introduced me to Allan Steinfeld, Nina Kuscsik, Grete Waitz, Sid Howard, and other legends at NYRR. Toshi lives on in all of us who were fortunate to know her. My years writing for *Runner's World* were a sportswriters' dream come true and I will be forever grateful to Amby Burfoot, Bart Yasso, Laurie Adams, and my editor Katie Neitz for their support and for opening up the door to the cadre of inspiring runners I wrote about over the years like Ed Whitlock, Ted Corbitt, Jamie and Lynn Parks, and others.

At New York Road Runners, huge thanks go to Gordon Bakoulis who brought me to NYRR after she left her role as editor of *Running Times*, where we first met. Stuart Calderwood, also a top NYRR editor and coach spent hours going through my copy to make sure my Ts were crossed and my Is were dotted. Gordon and Stuart helped with and encouraged this book. My NYRR Team for Kids teammates and co-workers are like family to me and further opened up a world of charity runners that became special to me through my years of coaching mostly first-time marathoners. Norm Solomon encouraged me to write this book saying, "We are all getting older and need the advice and inspiration."

Working at NYRR was a dream job and I can't quite cut that cord. There is nothing so rewarding as coaching first-time marathoners and see them cross the finish line in insurmountable joy at their achievement and getting lots of sweaty hugs.

I especially have to acknowledge all the people I profiled for this book. They opened up their lives to me and I am forever grateful to them. We laughed, we cried, and we talked about things I've been sworn to secrecy about. I hope to be like many of them as I go through the masters decades. Tom Perri and Ken Stone took time to help find me interesting people to write about and to fact check dates and times. A special thanks goes to Skyhorse Publishing who believed in this project and were super supportive throughout the creative process. My editor was patient with my (many) last minute changes and additions.

My husband Androc, and our kids, Elijah and Anna, continue to enrich my life. One more advantage to growing older is seeing our kids become responsible and loving adults, spouses and parents and people we want to hang out with. And now I have a granddaughter to teach to love running. Life just keeps getting better.